Plan Tasty Menus Easily With Good-for-You Foods!

By Diane Werner, Associate Food Editor and Registered Dietitian

SINCE the first edition of the *Down-Home Diabetic Cookbook* was published 5 years ago, we've received hundreds of letters from people thanking us for making it easy to create mouth-watering menus with restricted-diet recipes.

Most every letter ended with one simple request: "Could you *please* publish another book with dishes that are lower in sugar, salt and fat but yet full of flavor?"

We're happy to oblige! This second edition of the *Down-Home Diabetic Cookbook* features 300 country-style recipes that meet the needs of those on special diets. You're sure to love them just as much as—if not more than—the delicious dishes found in the first edition.

Many of the foods are "lighter" favorites of a particular cook's family. In other cases, our home economists have adjusted the ingredients of treasured recipes to meet the needs of those on restricted diets. Each and every recipe has been thoroughly tested in the Reiman Publications Test Kitchen and personally reviewed by me to ensure it meets all the qualifications required of a special-diet recipe.

For many years, I taught people with diabetes the importance of proper nutrition and also managed cafeterias in medical clinics and senior centers. So I know just how challenging it can be to come up with tasty, healthy foods day in and day out.

That's why I'm so thrilled about this second edition of the *Down-Home Diabetic Cookbook*. With 300 delicious recipes, you can create a new dish almost every day for a year! From Italian Beef Sandwiches, Blue-Ribbon Herb Rolls and Smoked Tenderloin Salad to Lemon Asparagus Soup, Chocolate Mousse with Strawberries and Icebox Sandwiches (a personal favorite of mine!), this recipe-packed book will appeal to *everyone* in the family, not just those on special diets.

Here are a few other things to keep in mind about this one-of-a-kind cookbook:

● Every recipe includes nutritional analysis and diabetic exchanges. Exchanges are based on the standards set by the American Diabetes Association and the American Dietetic Association.

● Although most recipes call for reduced-sodium canned products, they still deliver superior flavor. However, if you don't need to regulate your sodium intake, you may choose to use regular canned products.

● Whenever sugar is used in a recipe in this cookbook, it's included in the carbohydrate value used to calculate the diabetic exchange.

● If you have any questions about using sugar, or any other questions about your diet, special restrictions and how the recipes in this book fit into your individual program, contact your doctor or dietitian.

Who says you have to forgo flavor on a restricted diet? This *Down-Home Diabetic Cookbook* deliciously proves otherwise!

CONTENTS

Editor: Julie Schnittka
Food Editor: Janaan Cunningham
Associate Food Editor/Dietitian: Diane Werner, R.D.
Recipe Editor: Janet Briggs
Art Director: Ellen Lloyd
Associate Editors: Kristine Krueger, Heidi Lloyd
Test Kitchen Assistant: Suzanne Hampton
Food Photography Artist: Stephanie Marchese
Photo Studio Manager: Anne Schimmel
Illustrations: Jim Sibilski

©2000, Reiman Publications, LLC
5400 S. 60th Street, Greendale WI 53129
International Standard Book Number 0-89821-292-8
Library of Congress Control Card Number: 00-132685
All rights reserved. Printed in U.S.A.

PICTURED ON FRONT COVER: Peppered Beef Tenderloin (p. 123),
Broccoli Tomato Salad (p. 69) and Sherbet Cake Roll (p. 293).

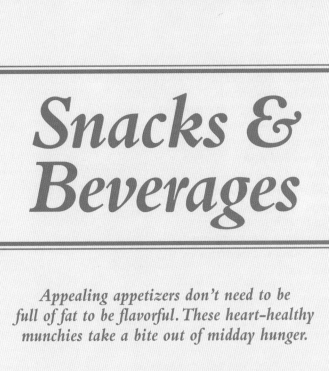

Snacks &
Beverages

*Appealing appetizers don't need to be
full of fat to be flavorful. These heart-healthy
munchies take a bite out of midday hunger.*

Vegetable Pizza

Marcia Tiernan, Madrid, New York

My sister brought this recipe with her when she was visiting from California. We served it at a family get-together and everyone just loved it. We're often asked to bring it to potlucks.

3 tubes (8 ounces *each*) reduced-
   fat refrigerated crescent rolls
2 packages (8 ounces *each*)
   fat-free cream cheese, softened
2/3 cup fat-free mayonnaise
1 tablespoon dill weed
4 tomatoes, seeded and
   chopped
2 cups chopped fresh broccoli
3 green onions, thinly sliced
2 cups sliced fresh mushrooms
1/2 medium green pepper, chopped
1 can (2-1/4 ounces) sliced ripe
   olives, drained
2 cups (8 ounces) fat-free
   shredded cheddar cheese

Unroll crescent roll dough and place in two 15-in. x 10-in. x 1-in. baking pans coated with nonstick cooking spray. Flatten dough, sealing seams and perforations. Bake at 400° for 10 minutes or until light golden brown. Cool. In a small bowl, blend cream cheese, mayonnaise and dill. Spread over crusts. Top with vegetables, olives and cheese. Cut into bite-size squares. Refrigerate until ready to serve. **Yield:** 96 servings.

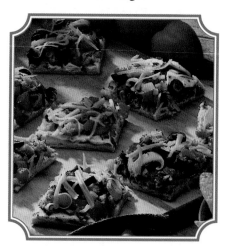

Exchanges: 1/2 Lean Meat, 1/2 Vegetable
Nutritional Information

Serving Size: 2 pieces
Calories: 79
Sodium: 235 mg
Cholesterol: 2 mg

Carbohydrate: 9 gm
Protein: 4 gm
Fat: 3 gm
Fiber: trace

Raspberry Cooler

DeAnn Alleva, Hudson, Wisconsin

*Here's a refreshing cooler for a late-summer afternoon.
This beverage is so pretty in a clear sparkling glass!*

**1 pint (2 cups) fresh *or* frozen
  unsweetened raspberries
4 cups light raspberry-cranberry
  juice
Mint sprigs, optional**

In a bowl, crush berries. Add juice and mix well. Strain through a fine sieve or cheesecloth. Refrigerate. Garnish with mint sprigs if desired. **Yield:** about 5 cups.

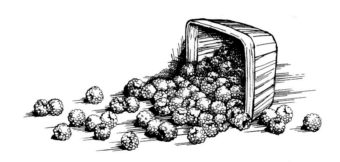

Exchanges: 1/2 Fruit
Nutritional Information

Serving Size: 1 cup
Calories: 60
Sodium: 4 mg
Cholesterol: 0 mg

Carbohydrate: 15 gm
Protein: trace
Fat: trace
Fiber: 3 gm

Creamy Dill Dip

Kathy Beldorth, Three Oaks, Michigan

Be prepared—you'll likely need to make a double batch of this delightful dip. One is never enough when we have a get-together. It tastes great with just about any vegetable, so you can use whatever you have on hand as dippers.

1 cup fat-free mayonnaise
1 cup (8 ounces) light sour cream
2 tablespoons dried parsley flakes
1 tablespoon dried minced onion
2 teaspoons dill weed
1-1/2 teaspoons salt-free seasoning
    blend
1 teaspoon sugar

In a small bowl, combine all ingredients. Chill for at least 1 hour. Serve with fresh vegetables or crackers. **Yield:** 2 cups.

SPREAD FOR BREAD. Creamy Dill Dip is also delicious spread on slices of whole wheat, rye or pumpernickel bread.

Exchanges: 1 Vegetable

Nutritional Information

Serving Size: 2 tablespoons
Calories: 33
Sodium: 117 mg
Cholesterol: 5 mg

Carbohydrate: 4 gm
Protein: 1 gm
Fat: 1 gm
Fiber: trace

Fresh Salsa

Terry Thompson, Albuquerque, New Mexico

After the mild green chilies I grow in my garden are roasted, I peel, dice and freeze them to use all year. This colorful salsa is a favorite.

6 Anaheim chilies, roasted, peeled and diced
4 large tomatoes, chopped
3 green onions, sliced
2 tablespoons minced fresh cilantro *or* parsley
1/2 to 1 jalapeno pepper, seeded and minced*
1 garlic clove, minced
1/3 cup cider *or* red wine vinegar
1/3 cup olive *or* vegetable oil
1/2 teaspoon pepper
1 teaspoon salt

In a bowl, combine chilies, tomatoes, onions, cilantro, jalapeno and garlic. In another bowl, combine vinegar, oil, pepper and salt; stir into vegetable mixture. Cover and chill for at least 2 hours. Serve with baked tortilla chips. **Yield:** 4-1/2 cups. ***Editor's Note:** When cutting or seeding hot peppers, use rubber gloves to protect your hands. Avoid touching your face.

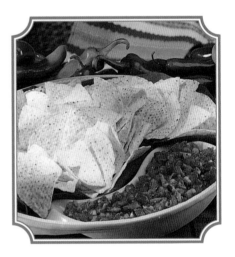

Exchanges: Free food

Nutritional Information

Serving Size: 2 tablespoons
Calories: 24
Sodium: 91 mg
Cholesterol: 0 mg

Carbohydrate: 1 gm
Protein: trace
Fat: 2 gm
Fiber: trace

Tasty Pork Nuggets

Katie Koziolek, Hartland, Minnesota

Through my many years of being married to a pork producer, I've come across quite a few wonderful recipes. These nuggets are fabulous finger food for snacks, lunches and dinners.

1 cup cornflake crumbs
1/3 cup toasted wheat germ
3 tablespoons sesame seeds
1-1/2 teaspoons dried parsley flakes
1/2 teaspoon paprika
1/2 teaspoon ground mustard
1/2 teaspoon celery salt
1/2 teaspoon onion powder
1/4 teaspoon salt-free lemon-pepper seasoning
1/4 teaspoon salt-free seasoning blend
1 pound lean boneless pork, cut into 1-inch x 1-1/2-inch cubes
1 cup plain nonfat yogurt

In a shallow bowl, combine the first 10 ingredients. Dip pork cubes in yogurt, then roll in crumb mixture. Arrange in a single layer in a shallow baking pan coated with nonstick cooking spray. Bake at 400° for 15-18 minutes or until juices run clear. For a crispier coating, broil for 2-3 minutes after baking. **Yield:** 2-1/2 dozen.

Exchanges: 1-1/2 Lean Meat, 1/2 Starch
Nutritional Information

Serving Size: 3 pieces
Calories: 129
Sodium: 217 mg
Cholesterol: 30 mg

Carbohydrate: 11 gm
Protein: 13 gm
Fat: 3 gm
Fiber: trace

Pineapple Cream Cheese Spread

Rita Addicks, Weimar, Texas

*With a refreshing pineapple taste,
this spread is satisfying and easy to make.
Try it on celery sticks or reduced-fat crackers.*

**1 package (8 ounces) fat-free
 cream cheese, softened**
**1 can (8 ounces) unsweetened
 crushed pineapple, drained**

In a bowl, combine cream cheese and pineapple. Serve with celery sticks or crackers. Store in the refrigerator. **Yield:** 1-1/8 cups.

CARING FOR CREAM CHEESE. Store cream cheese in its original packaging in the coldest part of the refrigerator. After opening, rewrap leftovers tightly in plastic wrap. Refrigerate and use within 1 week.

Exchanges: 1 Vegetable

Nutritional Information

Serving Size: 2 tablespoons
Calories: 32
Sodium: 138 mg
Cholesterol: 2 mg

Carbohydrate: 4 gm
Protein: 4 gm
Fat: trace
Fiber: trace

Tomato Chili Dip

Rachael Santarsiero, Orange City, Iowa

This fresh–tasting dip is excellent for summer barbecues and picnics. I like to use homegrown tomatoes for maximum flavor.

4 large ripe tomatoes
8 green onions
2 cans (4 ounces *each*) chopped green chilies
1 can (4-1/4 ounces) chopped ripe olives, drained
6 tablespoons cider *or* red wine vinegar
1 tablespoon olive *or* vegetable oil
1-1/2 to 2 teaspoons garlic powder
1 jalapeno pepper, seeded and minced*

Chop tomatoes and onions into 1/4-in. pieces; place in a large bowl. Stir in the next five ingredients. Add jalapeno. Cover and refrigerate overnight. Serve with baked tortilla chips. **Yield:** 8 cups. ***Editor's Note:** When cutting or seeding hot peppers, use rubber gloves to protect your hands. Avoid touching your face.

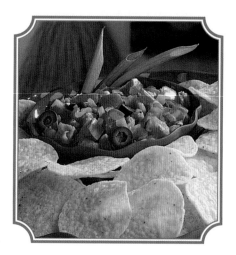

Exchanges: 1 Vegetable

Nutritional Information

Serving Size: 1/4 cup
Calories: 32
Sodium: 63 mg
Cholesterol: 0 mg

Carbohydrate: 2 gm
Protein: trace
Fat: trace
Fiber: trace

Tex-Mex Dip and Chips

Carol Battle, Heathsville, Virginia

For a cool, creamy snack with a bit of a kick, this recipe fits the bill. Amazingly, the dip has only two ingredients, and the baked pita bread "chips" are easy to make.

2 cups (16 ounces) nonfat sour cream
1 cup salsa
8 pita breads (6 inches)

In a bowl, combine sour cream and salsa. Cover and chill for at least 2 hours. Cut each pita into six wedges; separate each wedge into two pieces. Place on an ungreased baking sheet. Bake at 275° for 5-10 minutes or until crisp. Serve with the dip. **Yield:** 3 cups dip and 96 chips

ADD ZIP TO CHIPS. For added flavor, season the pita breads for Tex-Mex Dip and Chips with your family's favorite herbs or salt-free seasoning blend before baking as directed.

Exchanges: 1 Starch
Nutritional Information

Serving Size: 2 tablespoons dip and 4 chips
Calories: 83
Sodium: 197 mg
Cholesterol: 2 mg

Carbohydrate: 16 gm
Protein: 3 gm
Fat: trace
Fiber: 1 gm

Smokehouse Quesadillas

Sherri Winters, Trenton, Texas

Quesadillas are a nice alternative to traditional sandwiches. But our teenage children have also been known to eat them for breakfast!

1/4 cup fat-free ranch salad dressing
6 flour tortillas (7 inches)
6 thin slices (1 ounce *each*) fully cooked low-sodium ham
6 thin slices (1 ounce *each*) Monterey Jack cheese
3/4 cup salsa

Spread about 2 teaspoons of dressing on each tortilla. Top each with a slice of ham and a slice of cheese. Roll up jelly-roll style. In a nonstick skillet coated with nonstick cooking spray, cook quesadillas over medium heat, turning constantly, until cheese is melted. Cut each quesadilla into four pieces. Serve with salsa for dipping. **Microwave Directions:** Assemble quesadillas as directed. Wrap each quesadilla in paper towel and microwave on high for 1 minute or until cheese is melted. This recipe was tested in a 700-watt microwave. **Yield:** 2 dozen.

Exchanges: 1 Starch, 1/2 Meat

Nutritional Information

Serving Size: 2 pieces with 1 tablespoon salsa
Calories: 162
Sodium: 480 mg
Cholesterol: 23 mg

Carbohydrate: 16 gm
Protein: 8 gm
Fat: 7 gm
Fiber: trace

Cucumber Dill Spread

Doris Heath, Bryson City, North Carolina

*This creamy spread is so good on a hot summer day
served with an assortment of fresh vegetables or reduced-fat crackers.*

**2 packages (8 ounces *each*) fat-free
  cream cheese, softened**
2 teaspoons lemon juice
2 teaspoons minced onion
1/2 teaspoon dill weed
1/4 teaspoon prepared horseradish
1/8 teaspoon hot pepper sauce
3/4 cup finely diced seeded cucumber

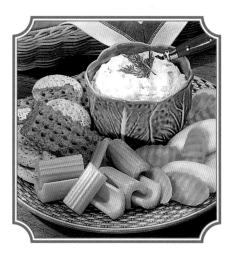

In a mixing bowl, beat cream cheese until smooth. Add lemon juice, onion, dill, horseradish and hot pepper sauce. Fold in cucumber. Cover and chill for at least 1 hour. Serve with fresh vegetables or crackers. **Yield:** 2-1/3 cups.

Exchanges: 1/2 Vegetable

Nutritional Information

Serving Size: 2 tablespoons
Calories: 25
Sodium: 139 mg
Cholesterol: 2 mg

Carbohydrate: 2 gm
Protein: 4 gm
Fat: trace
Fiber: trace

Morning Fruit Shake

Janet Kowalski, Brookfield, Wisconsin

In addition to offering an assortment of juices and milk, why not serve this refreshing beverage filled with your family's favorite fruit flavors? Your thirsty clan will savor it so much, you'll be asked to make it from sunrise to sundown!

1 cup light cranberry juice
2 medium ripe bananas, sliced
2 cartons (8 ounces *each*) light nonfat raspberry yogurt *or* flavor of choice
Sugar substitute equivalent to 1 tablespoon sugar
Few drops red food coloring, optional
Fresh raspberries, optional

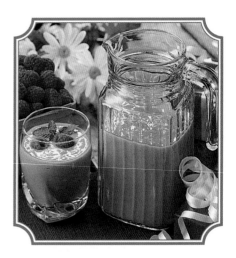

In a blender, combine the first five ingredients; cover and blend at medium speed until smooth. Serve immediately. Garnish with raspberries if desired. **Yield:** 4 servings.

Exchanges: 2 Fruit, 1/2 Skim Milk

Nutritional Information

Serving Size: 3/4 cup
Calories: 184
Sodium: 61 mg
Cholesterol: 9 mg

Carbohydrate: 39 gm
Protein: 5 gm
Fat: 1 gm
Fiber: 0 gm
(Calculated without garnish)

Party Pitas

Janette Root, Ellensburg, Washington

Whenever the ladies of our church host a bridal shower, these pita sandwiches appear on the menu. Not only are they easy and delicious, they add color to the table.

1 package (8 ounces) fat-free
   cream cheese, softened
1/2 cup fat-free mayonnaise
1/2 teaspoon dill weed
1/4 teaspoon garlic salt
 8 mini pita breads (4 inches)
16 fresh spinach leaves
3/4 pound shaved fully cooked
   low-sodium ham
1/2 pound thinly sliced reduced-fat
   Monterey Jack cheese

Combine cream cheese, mayonnaise, dill and garlic salt. Cut each pita in half horizontally; spread 1 tablespoon cream cheese mixture on cut sides. On eight pita halves, layer spinach, ham and cheese. Top with remaining pita halves. Cut each pita into four wedges; secure with a toothpick. **Yield:** 16 servings.

SPINACH STORAGE. Wash and dry fresh spinach thoroughly, removing stems. Wrap loosely in paper towels, store tightly sealed in a plastic bag and refrigerate for up to 3 days.

Exchanges: 1-1/2 Lean Meat, 1/2 Starch
Nutritional Information

Serving Size: 2 pieces
Calories: 126
Sodium: 546 mg
Cholesterol: 23 mg

Carbohydrate: 10 gm
Protein: 13 gm
Fat: 4 gm
Fiber: trace

Hawaiian Pizza

Gena Kuntz, West Springfield, Pennsylvania

When a friend ordered this pizza in a restaurant, I was skeptical. But after trying a slice, I was hooked! My family is thrilled that I serve this at least twice a month.

1 package (1/4 ounce) active dry yeast
1-1/4 cups warm water (110° to 115°)
3 to 3-1/4 cups all-purpose flour
1 tablespoon sugar
1 teaspoon salt
1 can (15 ounces) pizza sauce
3 cups (12 ounces) reduced-fat shredded mozzarella cheese
1 cup diced fully cooked low-sodium ham
1 can (8 ounces) unsweetened pineapple tidbits, drained

In a large mixing bowl, dissolve yeast in water. Add 1-1/2 cups flour, sugar and salt; beat until smooth. Add enough remaining flour to form a soft dough. Turn onto a floured surface; knead until smooth and elastic, about 6-8 minutes. Place in a greased bowl, turning once to grease top. Cover and let rise in a warm place until doubled, about 1 hour. Punch dough down; press onto the bottom and up the sides of a 15-in. x 10-in. x 1-in. baking pan coated with nonstick cooking spray. Spread with pizza sauce; sprinkle with cheese, ham and pineapple. Bake at 400° for 20-25 minutes or until the crust is browned and cheese is melted. Cut into bite-size squares and serve immediately. **Yield:** 48 servings.

Exchanges: 1 Starch, 1 Lean Meat

Nutritional Information

Serving Size: 2 pieces
Calories: 120
Sodium: 262 mg
Cholesterol: 13 mg

Carbohydrate: 16 gm
Protein: 8 gm
Fat: 3 gm
Fiber: 1 gm

Yogurt Fruit Dip

Sandy Szwarc, Albuquerque, New Mexico

Paired with an assortment of fresh fruit, this creamy dip is super for warm weather and nice enough for a special brunch.

1 carton (16 ounces) plain nonfat yogurt
2 tablespoons brown sugar
1 tablespoon orange juice concentrate
Dash ground cinnamon

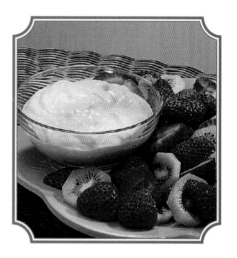

Line a strainer with a paper coffee filter or cheesecloth; place over a bowl. Put yogurt in strainer; refrigerate for 8 hours. Discard liquid in bowl. Combine yogurt, brown sugar, orange juice concentrate and cinnamon; mix well. Serve with fresh fruit.
Yield: 1-1/4 cups.

Exchanges: 1/2 Skim Milk

Nutritional Information

Serving Size: 2 tablespoons
Calories: 36
Sodium: 36 mg
Cholesterol: trace

Carbohydrate: 6 gm
Protein: 3 gm
Fat: trace
Fiber: 0 gm

Low-Fat Bean Dip

Gladys DeBoer, Castleford, Idaho

Whether you're hosting a party or just treating yourself, this creamy dip is great to snack on with fresh vegetables or baked tortilla chips.

3 tablespoons lemon juice
1 can (15 ounces) pinto beans, rinsed and drained
3 tablespoons chopped green onions
2 tablespoons fat-free mayonnaise
1-1/2 teaspoons seeded minced jalapeno pepper*
1 teaspoon Worcestershire sauce
1/2 teaspoon salt-free seasoning blend
1/4 teaspoon sugar

Combine all ingredients in a blender or food processor; cover and process until smooth. Transfer to a serving bowl. Serve with fresh vegetables or baked tortilla chips. Store in the refrigerator. **Yield:** 1-3/4 cups. **Editor's Note:** When cutting or seeding hot peppers, use rubber gloves to protect your hands. Avoid touching your face.

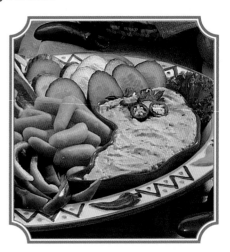

Exchanges: 1/2 Starch
Nutritional Information

Serving Size: 2 tablespoons
Calories: 42
Sodium: 153 mg
Cholesterol: 0 mg

Carbohydrate: 8 gm
Protein: 2 gm
Fat: trace
Fiber: 2 gm

Citrus Mint Punch

Judith Anglen, Riverton, Wyoming

Mint gives this citrus punch some real spark. I especially like to serve this beverage at bridal and baby showers and during the summer months at luncheons.

1 cup packed fresh mint leaves
Grated peel of 1 orange
Grated peel of 1 lemon
3 cups boiling water
1 can (12 ounces) frozen lemonade concentrate, thawed
1 can (12 ounces) frozen unsweetened orange juice concentrate, thawed
1-1/2 quarts cold water
Additional mint leaves, optional

Place mint and peels in a heat-resistant pitcher or bowl; add boiling water. Let steep for 1 hour; strain. Add concentrates and water; stir well. Refrigerate. Serve over ice; garnish with mint if desired. **Yield:** 18 servings (3 quarts).

> **MIND YOUR MINT.** Fresh herbs are very perishable, so buy only as much as you need. Immerse freshly cut stems in about 2 inches of water. Cover the leaves loosely with a plastic bag and refrigerate for a few days.

Exchanges: 1 Fruit

Nutritional Information

Serving Size: 2/3 cup
Calories: 67
Sodium: 2 mg
Cholesterol: 0 mg

Carbohydrate: 17 gm
Protein: trace
Fat: trace
Fiber: trace

Diabetic Milk Shake

Evelyn Archer, Elkville, Illinois

My husband could drink this beverage every day and never tire of it. It has just the right amount of sweetness.

3/4 cup fat-free sugar-free vanilla ice cream
3/4 cup skim milk
1 large ripe banana, quartered
Sugar substitute equivalent to 4 teaspoons sugar
1/8 teaspoon vanilla extract

Combine all ingredients in a blender; cover and process on low speed until smooth. Serve immediately. **Yield:** 2 servings.

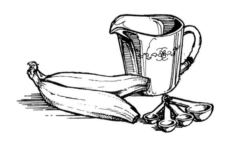

Exchanges: 1 Starch, 1 Fruit

Nutritional Information

Serving Size: 1 cup
Calories: 148
Sodium: 99 mg
Cholesterol: 2 mg

Carbohydrate: 32 gm
Protein: 7 gm
Fat: trace
Fiber: 1 gm

Veggie Christmas Tree

Leola Seltmann, Wichita, Kansas

*Flavor the holidays with this pretty and festive vegetable appetizer.
It's a "must make" at our house each Christmas!*

**1 bottle (8 ounces) fat-free ranch
  salad dressing**
4 cups broccoli florets
1 broccoli stem
3 to 4 cups cauliflowerets
**4 to 5 cherry tomatoes,
  quartered**
1 medium carrot, sliced

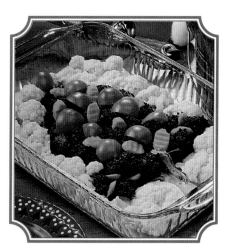

Cover the bottom of a 13-in. x 9-in. x 2-
in. glass dish with dressing. Arrange broccoli in a tree shape, using the stem as the
trunk. Place cauliflower around tree. Add
tomatoes and carrot slices as ornaments.
Yield: 20 servings.

Exchanges: 1 Vegetable
Nutritional Information
Serving Size: 1/20 recipe
Calories: 26
Sodium: 108 mg
Cholesterol: 0 mg

Carbohydrate: 6 gm
Protein: 1 gm
Fat: trace
Fiber: trace

Cajun Pork Sandwiches

Mae Kruse, Monee, Illinois

This recipe's specially seasoned rub gives tender juicy pork a slightly spicy flavor. You'll watch in delight as these delicious sandwiches disappear from your buffet table! I also like to prepare these for weekend lunches.

2 pork tenderloins (1 pound **each**), trimmed
2 teaspoons vegetable oil
3 tablespoons paprika
2 teaspoons dried oregano
2 teaspoons dried thyme
1-1/2 teaspoons garlic powder
1/2 teaspoon pepper
1/2 teaspoon salt-free seasoning blend
1/2 teaspoon ground cumin
1/4 teaspoon ground nutmeg
1/4 teaspoon cayenne pepper
36 French bread slices (3/4 inch thick)
3/4 cup fat-free mayonnaise
Lettuce leaves
Thin slivers of green and sweet red pepper

Place tenderloins in a 13-in. x 9-in. x 2-in. baking pan coated with nonstick cooking spray. Rub each with 1 teaspoon oil. In a bowl, combine seasonings; pat over tenderloins. Cover and refrigerate overnight. Bake at 425° for 25-30 minutes or until a meat thermometer reads 160°-170°. Let stand for 10 minutes; thinly slice. Spread bread with mayonnaise; top with lettuce, pork and peppers. **Yield:** 3 dozen.

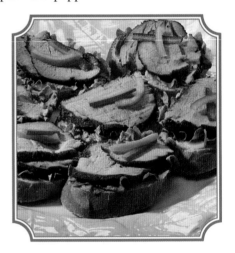

Exchanges: 1 Lean Meat, 1 Starch

Nutritional Information

Serving Size: 1 sandwich
Calories: 104
Sodium: 200 mg
Cholesterol: 16 mg

Carbohydrate: 14 gm
Protein: 7 gm
Fat: 2 gm
Fiber: trace

Herbed Vegetable Dip

Hazel Baber, Yuma, Arizona

*I like to keep this good-for-you dip on hand, along with a
variety of cut-up vegetables, for an easy snack.*

1 carton (16 ounces) low-fat
  cottage cheese
3 tablespoons skim milk
3/4 cup fat-free mayonnaise
1 tablespoon dried minced
  onion
1 tablespoon dried parsley
  flakes
1 teaspoon dill weed
1 teaspoon salt-free seasoning
  blend
1/4 teaspoon garlic powder

In a blender, blend cottage cheese and
milk until smooth. Stir in remaining ingredients and mix well. Chill overnight.
Serve with fresh vegetables or crackers.
Yield: 2-1/2 cups.

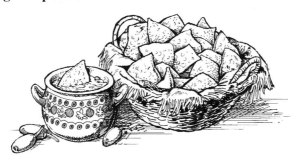

Exchanges: Free food
Nutritional Information

Serving Size: 2 tablespoons
Calories: 28
Sodium: 157 mg
Cholesterol: 2 mg

Carbohydrate: 2 gm
Protein: 3 gm
Fat: trace
Fiber: trace

Icebox Sandwiches

Sandy Armijo, Naples, Italy

My mother liked making these cool creamy treats when I was growing up in the States because they're so quick to fix. Now my three kids enjoy them.

2 cups cold skim milk
1 package (1 ounce) instant
   sugar-free vanilla pudding mix
2 cups light whipped topping
3/4 cup miniature semisweet
   chocolate chips
1/2 teaspoon vanilla extract
42 reduced-fat graham cracker
   squares

Mix milk and pudding according to package directions and refrigerate until set. Fold in whipped topping, chocolate chips and vanilla. Place 21 graham crackers on a baking sheet; top each with about 3 tablespoons filling. Place another graham cracker on top. Freeze for 1 hour or until firm. Wrap individually in plastic wrap; freeze. Serve sandwiches frozen. **Yield:** 21 sandwiches.

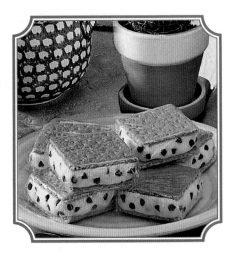

Exchanges: 1 Starch, 1/2 Fat

Nutritional Information

Serving Size: 1 sandwich
Calories: 114
Sodium: 125 mg
Cholesterol: trace

Carbohydrate: 19 gm
Protein: 2 gm
Fat: 3 gm
Fiber: 1 gm

Hearty Salads

When you're in the mood for a little lighter fare for lunch or dinner, toss together a scrumptious salad loaded with meats, vegetables, pasta and more.

Spicy Beef Salad

Peggy Allen, Pasadena, California

This pretty salad is fast to prepare after a long day at work.

1/3 cup lime juice
 1 tablespoon brown sugar
 1 tablespoon light soy sauce
 1 tablespoon minced fresh
   basil *or* 1 teaspoon dried basil
 2 teaspoons minced fresh mint
   or 3/4 teaspoon dried mint
 1 jalapeno pepper, minced*
 2 to 3 garlic cloves, minced
 1 teaspoon grated fresh
   gingerroot *or* 1/4 to 1/2
   teaspoon ground ginger
1/2 pound boneless sirloin steak,
   thinly sliced
 1 large sweet red pepper,
   julienned
1/2 medium cucumber, chopped
 6 cups torn mixed salad greens

For dressing, combine the first five ingredients; set aside. In a medium nonstick skillet coated with nonstick cooking spray, saute jalapeno, garlic and ginger for 30 seconds. Add beef; stir-fry until cooked as desired. Remove from the heat. Add red pepper and cucumber; toss gently. Place greens on a serving plate; top with beef mixture. Add dressing to pan and bring to a boil; drizzle over salad. Serve immediately. **Yield:** 4 servings. ***Editor's Note:** When cutting or seeding hot peppers, use rubber gloves to protect your hands. Avoid touching your face.

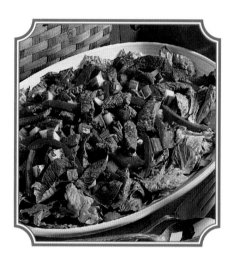

Exchanges: 2 Lean Meat, 1 Vegetable

Nutritional Information

Serving Size: 1/4 recipe
Calories: 127
Sodium: 285 mg
Cholesterol: 33 mg

Carbohydrate: 11 gm
Protein: 14 gm
Fat: 3 gm
Fiber: 2 gm

Grill-Side Turkey Salad

Barbara Young, Bethesda, Maryland

*I've enjoyed cooking for as long as I can remember...I even
majored in home economics in college. I now
enthusiastically cook and bake with my granddaughter.*

2 turkey breast tenderloins
  (1-1/2 pounds)
2 teaspoons dried tarragon,
  divided
1/2 cup thinly sliced celery
1/2 cup chopped green pepper
1/2 cup chopped red onion
  2 tablespoons vegetable oil
1 tablespoon light soy sauce
1 tablespoon lemon juice
1 tablespoon cider *or* red
  wine vinegar
1/8 teaspoon pepper
1/4 teaspoon salt-free seasoning
  blend
Lettuce leaves

Sprinkle each tenderloin with 1/2 teaspoon tarragon. Grill, uncovered, over medium-hot heat for 8-10 minutes on each side or until a meat thermometer reads 170°-180°. Cool to room temperature. Cut into cubes; place in a large bowl. Add celery, green pepper and onion. In a small bowl, combine oil, soy sauce, lemon juice, vinegar, pepper, seasoning blend and remaining tarragon; mix well. Pour over turkey mixture; toss to coat. Refrigerate for at least 3 hours. Serve on lettuce. **Yield:** 5 servings.

Exchanges: 4-1/2 Lean Meat, 1/2 Vegetable

Nutritional Information

Serving Size: 1/5 recipe
Calories: 212
Sodium: 259 mg
Cholesterol: 84 mg

Carbohydrate: 3 gm
Protein: 34 gm
Fat: 6 gm
Fiber: trace

Turkey-Blue Cheese Pasta Salad

Angela Leinenbach, Newport News, Virginia

The blue cheese dressing makes this pasta salad unique and delicious. I've served it many times, and it's always a hit.

1 box (16 ounces) pasta shells, cooked, drained and cooled
3 cups cubed cooked turkey *or* chicken breast
1 cup diced green pepper
1/4 cup chopped onion
1 cup fat-free blue cheese salad dressing
1/4 cup nonfat sour cream

2 teaspoons celery seed
1/2 teaspoon salt-free seasoning blend
1/4 teaspoon pepper

Combine pasta, turkey, green pepper and onion in a large bowl. In a small bowl, combine the remaining ingredients; pour over salad and toss. Serve immediately. **Yield:** 12 servings.

SAVOR SOUR CREAM. Nonfat sour cream is made from skim milk instead of cream, so you can avoid the fat naturally but still have terrific flavor.

Exchanges: 1-1/2 Lean Meat, 1/2 Starch

Nutritional Information

Serving Size: 1/12 recipe
Calories: 157
Sodium: 258 mg
Cholesterol: 30 mg

Carbohydrate: 21 gm
Protein: 14 gm
Fat: 2 gm
Fiber: 1 gm

Chicken and Black Bean Salad

Cindie Ekstrand, Duarte, California

Here in California, we cook out year-round. I grill extra chicken specifically for this quick meal. It's so colorful and fresh-tasting that even our kids love it.

1/3 cup olive *or* vegetable oil
2 tablespoons lime juice
2 tablespoons chopped fresh cilantro *or* parsley
1-1/2 teaspoons sugar
1 garlic clove, minced
1/2 teaspoon chili powder
1/2 teaspoon salt-free seasoning blend
1/4 teaspoon pepper
1 can (15 ounces) black beans, rinsed and drained
1 can (11 ounces) Mexicorn, drained
1 medium sweet red pepper, julienned
1/3 cup sliced green onions
6 cups torn romaine
1-1/2 cups cooked chicken breast strips
Additional cilantro *or* parsley, optional

In a jar with tight-fitting lid, combine the first eight ingredients; shake well and set aside. In a bowl, toss beans, corn, red pepper and onions. Arrange romaine on a serving plate; top with bean mixture and chicken. Drizzle with dressing; garnish with cilantro if desired. **Yield:** 6 servings.

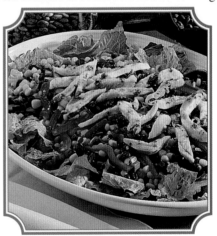

Exchanges: 1-1/2 Lean Meat, 1 Starch, 1 Fat, 1/2 Vegetable

Nutritional Information

Serving Size: 1/6 recipe
Calories: 290
Sodium: 540 mg
Cholesterol: 30 mg

Carbohydrate: 23 gm
Protein: 17 gm
Fat: 14 gm
Fiber: 6 gm

Summertime Main-Dish Salad

Ruby Williams, Bogalusa, Louisiana

*With a blend of ham, rice, vegetables and seasonings,
this cool and satisfying salad has all the spark of Cajun jambalaya.
It's a wonderful warm-weather meal.*

**2-1/2 cups cubed fully cooked
    low-sodium ham**
1/3 cup chopped onion
2 garlic cloves, minced
1 teaspoon dried oregano
1 teaspoon dried thyme
1/4 teaspoon cayenne pepper
1/4 teaspoon pepper
1 tablespoon vegetable oil
1/3 cup cider *or* red wine vinegar
4 cups cooked rice
3 cups diced cooked chicken
2 celery ribs, thinly sliced
1/2 cup julienned sweet red pepper
2 green onions with tops, sliced
1 pint cherry tomatoes

In a skillet over medium heat, saute the ham, onion and seasonings in oil until the onion is tender. Remove from the heat; stir in vinegar. Cool for 5 minutes. In a bowl, toss rice, chicken, celery, red pepper and green onions. Stir in the ham mixture. Cover and chill for at least 2 hours. Garnish with tomatoes. **Yield:** 9 servings.

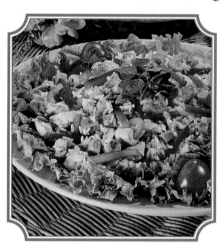

Exchanges: 3-1/2 Lean Meat, 1 Starch, 1 Vegetable

Nutritional Information

Serving Size: 1/9 recipe
Calories: 293
Sodium: 658 mg
Cholesterol: 73 mg

Carbohydrate: 25 gm
Protein: 30 gm
Fat: 7 gm
Fiber: 1 gm

Tropical Turkey Salad

Penny Gillard, San Antonio, Texas

*When my husband brought home a lunch guest unexpectedly
one day, I created this salad on the spot using leftover holiday turkey.
It's such a family favorite that I make it year-round.*

1 can (20 ounces) unsweetened
  pineapple tidbits
3 cups cubed cooked turkey breast
1 can (8 ounces) sliced water
  chestnuts, drained and halved
1 cup thinly sliced fresh
  mushrooms
1 cup thinly sliced celery
1/2 cup thinly sliced green onions
3/4 cup fat-free ranch salad
  dressing
1/8 teaspoon garlic powder
1/8 teaspoon onion powder
7 cups torn mixed greens
2 tablespoons slivered almonds,
  toasted

Drain pineapple, reserving 3 tablespoons juice. In a large bowl, combine pineapple, turkey, water chestnuts, mushrooms, celery and onions. In a small bowl, combine pineapple juice, dressing, garlic powder and onion powder. Add to turkey mixture; toss to coat. Divide greens among nine plates; top each with 1 cup turkey mixture. Sprinkle with almonds. **Yield:** 9 servings.

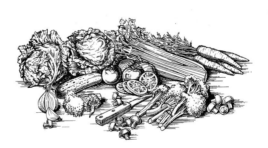

Exchanges: 2 Lean Meat, 1 Vegetable, 1/2 Fruit

Nutritional Information

Serving Size: 1/9 recipe
Calories: 165
Sodium: 61 mg
Cholesterol: 71 mg

Carbohydrate: 10 gm
Protein: 27 gm
Fat: 2 gm
Fiber: 2 gm

Basil Pasta and Ham Salad

Pauline Piggott, Northville, Michigan

With fresh basil and tomatoes in the dressing, this refreshing salad delightfully captures the flavor of summer.

TOMATO BASIL DRESSING:
- **1 cup chopped fresh tomatoes**
- **1/4 cup chopped fresh basil**
- **2 tablespoons chopped green onions**
- **2 tablespoons olive *or* vegetable oil**
- **2 tablespoons lemon juice**
- **1 garlic clove, minced**
- **1/2 teaspoon sugar**
- **1/4 teaspoon salt-free seasoning blend**
- **1/4 teaspoon pepper**

SALAD:
- **2-1/2 cups (10 ounces) uncooked spiral pasta**
- **1 cup cubed fully cooked low-sodium ham**
- **1 can (2-1/4 ounces) sliced ripe olives, drained**
- **1/3 cup chopped fresh basil**

In a small bowl, combine the dressing ingredients. Refrigerate for at least 15 minutes. Cook pasta according to package directions; drain and rinse with cold water. Place in a large bowl. Add ham, olives and basil; toss. Add dressing and toss to coat. **Yield:** 8 servings.

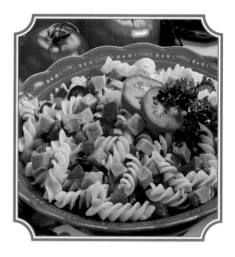

Exchanges: 1-1/2 Starch, 1 Lean Meat

Nutritional Information

Serving Size: 1/8 recipe
Calories: 208
Sodium: 349 mg
Cholesterol: 15 mg

Carbohydrate: 27 gm
Protein: 10 gm
Fat: 6 gm
Fiber: 2 gm

Chicken Salad Oriental

Vivian Miller, Sonora, California

Our family enjoys sampling a variety of salads, but this one is at the top of our list. It's an interesting twist on traditional chicken salad.

1-1/2 cups cubed cooked chicken breast
1-1/2 cups cooked rice
   1 package (10 ounces) frozen green beans, thawed
   1 cup fresh bean sprouts
   1 medium green pepper, chopped
   1 small onion, chopped
   2 tablespoons minced fresh parsley
DRESSING:
   1/3 cup nonfat sour cream
   2 tablespoons water
   2 tablespoons light soy sauce
   1/2 teaspoon garlic powder
   1/2 teaspoon salt-free seasoning blend
   1/4 teaspoon ground ginger
   1/8 teaspoon pepper

In a large bowl, combine the first seven ingredients. Whisk dressing ingredients together in a small bowl. Pour over salad; toss to coat. Refrigerate 8 hours or overnight. **Yield:** 6 servings.

BEAN SPROUT BASICS. Rinse fresh bean sprouts in cold water and pat dry. Place in a plastic bag with a dry paper towel and store in the refrigerator for up to 3 days. Rinse the sprouts again before using.

Exchanges: 1-1/2 Lean Meat, 1-1/2 Vegetable, 1/2 Starch

Nutritional Information

Serving Size: 1/6 recipe
Calories: 161
Sodium: 342 mg
Cholesterol: 31 mg

Carbohydrate: 22 gm
Protein: 15 gm
Fat: 2 gm
Fiber: 3 gm

Luncheon Pasta Salad

Julie Heitsch, St. Louis, Michigan

*I first tasted this salad at a ladies' luncheon at church.
My husband and children ask for this dish regularly.
Freshly baked breadsticks are a tasty accompaniment.*

1 cup spiral pasta, cooked,
 drained and cooled
1 cup cubed fully cooked
 low-sodium ham
1 small cucumber, diced
1 small tomato, seeded and diced
5 radishes, sliced
2 tablespoons diced onion
1 bottle (8 ounces) reduced-fat
 cucumber ranch salad dressing,
 divided
1/4 teaspoon salt-free seasoning
 blend

1/4 teaspoon pepper
4 cups torn lettuce
3/4 cup cubed reduced-fat cheddar
 cheese

In a large bowl, combine the first six ingredients. Add 1/2 cup dressing, seasoning blend and pepper; toss to coat. Cover and refrigerate for at least 2 hours. Just before serving, add lettuce, cheese and remaining dressing; toss. **Yield:** 8 servings.

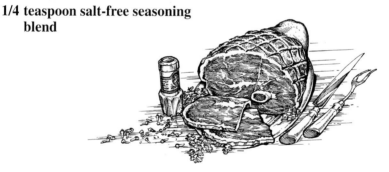

Exchanges: 1 Lean Meat, 1/2 Vegetable, 1/2 Starch

Nutritional Information

Serving Size: 1/8 recipe
Calories: 140
Sodium: 601 mg
Cholesterol: 17 mg

Carbohydrate: 18 gm
Protein: 11 gm
Fat: 3 gm
Fiber: 2 gm

Smoked Tenderloin Salad

Roberta Whitesell, Phoenix, Arizona

During our hot summers, I rely on salads to satisfy my family for lunch and dinner. In this recipe, the pork is grilled, so I can stay out of the kitchen.

DRESSING:
   1/2 cup orange juice
   2 tablespoons olive *or* vegetable oil
   2 tablespoons cider vinegar
   1 tablespoon grated orange peel
   2 teaspoons honey
   2 teaspoons Dijon mustard
   1/2 teaspoon coarsely ground pepper
SALAD:
   1 pork tenderloin (1 pound),
      trimmed
   10 cups torn salad greens
   2 seedless oranges, peeled and
      sectioned
   1/4 cup chopped pistachios

In a small bowl, combine the dressing ingredients; cover and chill. Grill pork, covered, over medium heat for 15-20 minutes or until a meat thermometer reads 160°-170°, turning occasionally. Let stand for 5 minutes; cut into thin slices. To serve, line a large platter with greens; top with orange sections and tenderloin. Sprinkle with pistachios. Drizzle with dressing. **Yield:** 5 servings.

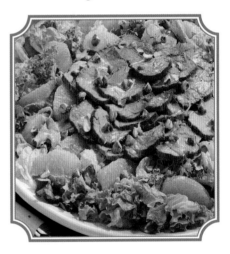

Exchanges: 2-1/2 Lean Meat, 1 Fruit, 1 Fat
Nutritional Information

Serving Size: 1/5 recipe
Calories: 244
Sodium: 125 mg
Cholesterol: 59 mg

Carbohydrate: 16 gm
Protein: 22 gm
Fat: 11 gm
Fiber: 4 gm

Warm Fajita Salad

Bobbie Jo Yokley, Franklin, Kentucky

This recipe earns rave reviews whenever I make it.

1 cup lime juice
1/4 cup low-sodium chicken broth
1/4 cup light soy sauce
2 garlic cloves, minced
1 tablespoon vegetable oil
1 teaspoon sugar
1 teaspoon liquid smoke
3/4 teaspoon ground cumin
1/2 teaspoon dried oregano
1/4 teaspoon ground ginger
1/4 teaspoon hot pepper sauce
1 pound boneless pork loin,
   trimmed and cut into thin strips
1 large onion, sliced
1 medium green pepper, cut into
   strips
1 medium sweet yellow pepper, cut
   into strips
1 tablespoon lemon juice
6 cups torn romaine
12 cherry tomatoes, quartered

In a large resealable plastic bag, combine the first 11 ingredients. Remove 2 tablespoons; cover and chill. Add pork to remaining marinade; toss to coat. Cover and chill for 30 minutes to 3 hours, turning occasionally. Drain pork, discarding marinade. Heat reserved marinade in a large skillet over medium-high heat. Add pork, onion and peppers; stir-fry for 3-4 minutes or until pork is no longer pink. Drizzle with lemon juice. Remove from the heat. Arrange romaine on five plates; top with meat mixture and tomatoes. **Yield:** 5 servings.

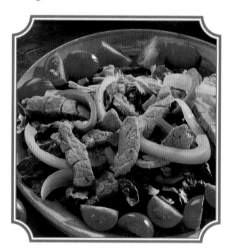

Exchanges: 2-1/2 Lean Meat, 1 Starch, 1 Vegetable, 1/2 Fat

Nutritional Information

Serving Size: 1/5 recipe
Calories: 278
Sodium: 555 mg
Cholesterol: 57 mg

Carbohydrate: 16 gm
Protein: 21 gm
Fat: 15 gm
Fiber: 3 gm

Greek Rice Salad

Barbara Nowakowski, North Tonawanda, New York

I love cooking. My husband even had to build another room especially for the cookbooks I collected! No matter how many salad recipes I try, this one is still at the top of my list.

4 cups cooked brown rice
2 cups julienned cooked turkey breast
2 cups halved cherry tomatoes
1 cup halved ripe olives
3/4 cup plain nonfat yogurt
3 to 4 tablespoons minced fresh mint
2 tablespoons cider *or* red wine vinegar
1/2 teaspoon salt-free lemon-pepper seasoning
1/4 cup crumbled feta cheese

In a large bowl, combine rice, turkey, tomatoes and olives. In a small bowl, combine yogurt, mint, vinegar and lemon pepper; mix well. Pour over rice mixture; toss to coat. Sprinkle with cheese. **Yield:** 8 servings.

FREEZING FETA CHEESE. Wrap leftover feta cheese tightly in freezer wrap and freeze for up to 2 months. Thaw in the refrigerator before using.

Exchanges: 2 Lean Meat, 1–1/2 Starch

Nutritional Information

Serving Size: 1 cup
Calories: 239
Sodium: 255 mg
Cholesterol: 52 mg

Carbohydrate: 28 gm
Protein: 22 gm
Fat: 4 gm
Fiber: 3 gm

Fruited Turkey Salad

Dorothy Rieke, Julian, Nebraska

*During my spare time, I can be found in the kitchen...
I love trying new recipes. In this turkey salad, fruit adds a
little sweetness while sunflower kernels add special crunch.*

4 cups cubed cooked turkey breast
1 can (20 ounces) unsweetened
  pineapple chunks, drained
1 cup seedless green grapes,
  halved
1 cup sliced celery
2 tablespoons vegetable oil
2 tablespoons orange juice
2 tablespoons lemon juice
1 tablespoon minced fresh parsley
1/2 teaspoon salt-free seasoning
  blend
1/2 cup fat-free mayonnaise
1/2 cup unsalted sunflower kernels

In a large bowl, combine turkey, pineapple, grapes and celery. Whisk together oil, orange juice, lemon juice, parsley and seasoning blend in a small bowl. Pour over salad; toss to coat. Refrigerate for 2 hours. Just before serving, add mayonnaise and sunflower kernels; mix well. **Yield:** 8 servings.

STORING SUNFLOWER KERNELS. Sunflower kernels (sunflower seeds without the shell) should be kept in an airtight container in the refrigerator or freezer for up to 1 year.

Exchanges: 4 Lean Meat, 1 Fat, 1/2 Fruit

Nutritional Information

Serving Size: 1/8 recipe
Calories: 282
Sodium: 179 mg
Cholesterol: 94 mg

Carbohydrate: 15 gm
Protein: 36 gm
Fat: 8 gm
Fiber: 2 gm

Pork 'n' Sweet Potato Salad

June Gerlach, St. Petersburg, Florida

*Instead of traditional salads that are tossed together,
this is layered for a beautiful presentation.
It's wonderful for special occasions.*

1 can (20 ounces) unsweeteneed
  pineapple chunks, undrained
1 cup fat-free mayonnaise
2 teaspoons curry powder
1/4 teaspoon paprika
1 small bunch romaine
2 pounds sweet potatoes, cooked,
  peeled and sliced
2 cups cubed cooked lean pork
1 medium green pepper, cut into
  chunks
1 small onion, minced
1/4 cup slivered almonds, toasted

Drain pineapple, reserving 3 tablespoons juice; set pineapple aside. Combine the juice, mayonnaise, curry powder and paprika. Line a large serving platter with romaine. Arrange potatoes, pork, pineapple, green pepper and onion on top. Sprinkle with almonds. Top with the dressing. **Yield:** 6 servings.

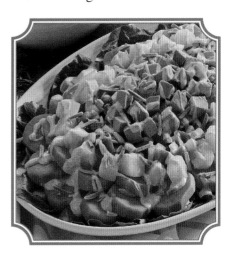

Exchanges: 2-1/2 Starch, 1-1/2 Lean Meat, 1 Vegetable, 1 Fat, 1/2 Fruit

Nutritional Information

Serving Size: 1/6 recipe
Calories: 366
Sodium: 329 mg
Cholesterol: 36 mg

Carbohydrate: 56 gm
Protein: 19 gm
Fat: 8 gm
Fiber: 8 gm

Grilled Chicken Salad

Brenda Eichelberger, Williamsport, Maryland

I frequently prepare this fabulous, filling salad for supper.

1 can (8 ounces) unsweetened
  sliced pineapple
3 tablespoons vegetable oil
2 tablespoons light soy sauce
1 tablespoon vinegar
1 tablespoon honey
1/4 teaspoon ground ginger
1/4 teaspoon cayenne pepper
4 boneless skinless chicken breast
  halves (1 pound)
1/2 to 1 teaspoon black pepper
5 cups torn salad greens
1 small green pepper, julienned
1 small sweet red pepper,
  julienned
1 cup sliced fresh mushrooms
1 small onion, sliced into rings

Drain pineapple, reserving 2 tablespoons juice. In a jar with tight-fitting lid, combine the juice, oil, soy sauce, vinegar, honey, ginger and cayenne; shake well. Brush some over pineapple slices; set aside. Sprinkle both sides of chicken with pepper; grill or broil for 4-5 minutes on each side or until juices run clear. Slice into strips. Grill or broil pineapple, turning to brown both sides, for 2-3 minutes or until heated through. Toss greens, peppers, mushrooms and onion in a large bowl; top with chicken and pineapple. Drizzle with remaining dressing. **Yield:** 4 servings.

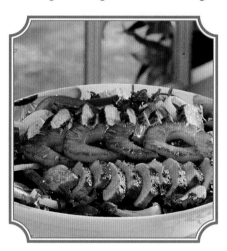

Exchanges: 3-1/2 Lean Meat, 2-1/2 Vegetable

Nutritional Information

Serving Size: 1/4 recipe
Calories: 331
Sodium: 551 mg
Cholesterol: 66 mg

Carbohydrate: 27 gm
Protein: 30 gm
Fat: 12 gm
Fiber: 4 gm

Salmon Salad

Diane Benskin, Lewisville, Texas

I'm an avid herb gardener and can't wait to use the products of my labor in dishes like this salad. For a different twist, I include chopped apple...it adds some natural sweetness.

2 cans (14-3/4 ounces *each*) salmon, drained and bones removed
2 celery ribs, sliced
1 large apple, peeled and chopped
5 green onions, sliced
1/2 cup fat-free mayonnaise
2 teaspoons snipped fresh dill *or* 3/4 teaspoon dill weed

3/4 teaspoon minced fresh basil *or* pinch dried basil
1/4 teaspoon garlic salt
1/4 teaspoon minced fresh tarragon *or* pinch dried tarragon

Flake salmon into a bowl. Add remaining ingredients; stir gently. Chill until ready to serve. **Yield:** 8 servings.

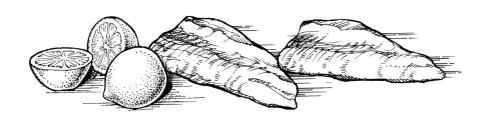

Exchanges: 3 Lean Meat

Nutritional Information

Serving Size: 1/2 cup
Calories: 178
Sodium: 681 mg
Cholesterol: 41 mg

Carbohydrate: 7 gm
Protein: 23 gm
Fat: 6 gm
Fiber: 1 gm

Refreshing Turkey Salad

Carolyn Lough, Medley, Alberta

When the heat of summer hits, I want to spend time with my family, not with my oven! So I'll often cook a turkey breast, then dice and freeze leftovers for fast hearty dishes like this.

3 cups cooked wild rice
2 cups cubed cooked turkey breast
2 cups thinly sliced celery
1/2 cup seedless green grapes, halved
1/2 cup seedless red grapes, halved
1/4 cup chopped green pepper
1/4 cup chopped sweet red pepper
1 jar (2 ounces) chopped pimientos, drained
1/2 cup fat-free mayonnaise
1/2 cup nonfat sour cream
1 tablespoon honey
1 teaspoon Dijon mustard
1 teaspoon celery seeds
1/2 teaspoon poppy seeds
1/2 teaspoon salt-free seasoning blend
1/4 teaspoon pepper
1 tablespoon slivered almonds, toasted

In a bowl, combine rice, turkey, celery, grapes, peppers and pimientos; set aside. In a small bowl, combine mayonnaise, sour cream, honey, mustard and seasonings; mix well. Pour over rice mixture; toss to coat. Cover and refrigerate for at least 1 hour. Sprinkle with almonds just before serving. **Yield:** 8 servings.

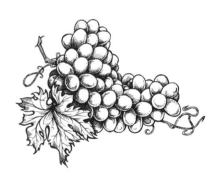

Exchanges: 1-1/2 Very Lean Meat, 1 Starch, 1/2 Fruit

Nutritional Information

Serving Size: 1/8 recipe
Calories: 203
Sodium: 209 mg
Cholesterol: 31 mg

Carbohydrate: 30 gm
Protein: 15 gm
Fat: 2 gm
Fiber: 2 gm

Layered Spinach Salad

Lori Cumberledge, Pasadena, Maryland

When this dish goes on a buffet, it's a real eye-catcher with its colorful layers. People enjoy the unique addition of cheese tortellini. This salad always goes fast!

1 package (9 ounces) refrigerated cheese tortellini
2 cups shredded red cabbage
6 cups torn fresh spinach
2 cups cherry tomatoes, halved
1/2 cup sliced green onions
1 bottle (8 ounces) fat-free ranch salad dressing
8 turkey bacon strips, cooked and crumbled

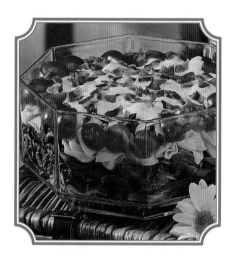

Cook tortellini according to package directions. Drain and rinse with cold water. In a large glass bowl, layer cabbage, spinach, tortellini, tomatoes and onions. Pour dressing over top; sprinkle with bacon. Cover and refrigerate for at least 1 hour. **Yield:** 10 servings.

Exchanges: 1 Starch, 1 Vegetable

Nutritional Information

Serving Size: 1/10 recipe
Calories: 162
Sodium: 453 mg
Cholesterol: 19 mg

Carbohydrate: 23 gm
Protein: 7 gm
Fat: 4 gm
Fiber: 2 gm

Curried Ham and Fruit Salad

Anne Frederick, New Hartford, New York

*This good-for-you salad is a quick and convenient
way to use up leftover ham. Plus, I've found
that it's perfect to serve as a special salad at luncheons.*

1-1/2 cups cubed fully cooked
    low-sodium ham
  2 medium red apples, cut into
    1/2-inch cubes
1/2 cup sliced celery
1/2 cup fat-free mayonnaise
  1 tablespoon skim milk
1/2 teaspoon curry powder
  1 small cantaloupe, cut into
    six wedges

In a large bowl, combine ham, apples and celery. In a small bowl, combine mayonnaise, milk and curry powder; pour over ham mixture and toss to coat. Cover and refrigerate for 1 hour. Serve over melon wedges. **Yield:** 6 servings.

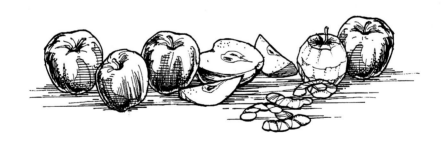

Exchanges: 1-1/2 Lean Meat, 1 Fruit, 1/2 Fat

Nutritional Information

Serving Size: 1/6 recipe
Calories: 173
Sodium: 716 mg
Cholesterol: 30 mg

Carbohydrate: 23 gm
Protein: 13 gm
Fat: 3 gm
Fiber: 3 gm

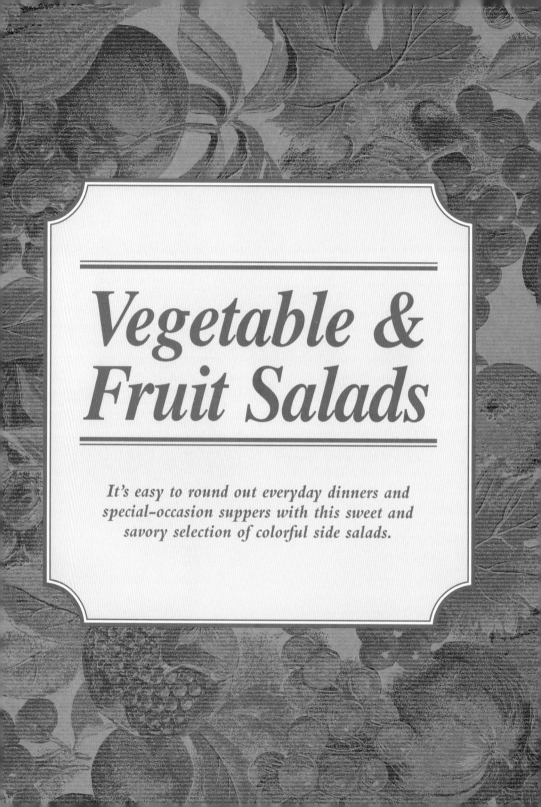

Vegetable & Fruit Salads

It's easy to round out everyday dinners and special-occasion suppers with this sweet and savory selection of colorful side salads.

Two-Bean Rice Salad

Lois Kodada, Northfield, Minnesota

*I've had many people tell me how much they like
this salad. It's a great dish to take to a potluck dinner.*

3 cups cooked wild rice
1 can (15 ounces) pinto beans,
  rinsed and drained
1 can (15 ounces) black beans,
  rinsed and drained
1 package (10 ounces) frozen
  peas, thawed
1 cup sliced celery
1 medium onion, chopped
1 can (4 ounces) chopped green
  chilies
1/4 cup chopped fresh parsley *or*
  cilantro
1/2 cup cider *or* white wine vinegar
1/4 cup olive *or* vegetable oil
2 tablespoons water
3/4 teaspoon salt-free seasoning
  blend
1/2 teaspoon garlic powder
1/2 teaspoon pepper

In a large salad bowl, combine the rice,
beans, peas, celery, onion, chilies and
parsley or cilantro; mix well. Combine the
remaining ingredients in a jar with tight-
fitting lid; shake well. Pour over rice mixture; toss to coat. Cover and refrigerate for
at least 1 hour. **Yield:** 18 servings.

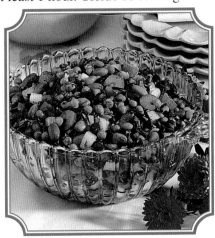

Exchanges: 1 Starch, 1/2 Fat

Nutritional Information

Serving Size: 1/2 cup
Calories: 121
Sodium: 118 mg
Cholesterol: 0 mg

Carbohydrate: 18 gm
Protein: 5 gm
Fat: 3 gm
Fiber: 5 gm

Molded Cranberry Fruit Salad

Virginia Rexroat, Jenks, Oklahoma

*Cooking for someone on a restricted diet can be a real challenge,
especially during the holidays when richer foods are prevalent.
This cool salad appeals to all palates.*

**2 packages (.6 ounce *each*) sugar-
free cherry gelatin**
2 cups boiling water
**1 bag (12 ounces) fresh *or* frozen
cranberries**
1 large apple, peeled and chopped
**1 large orange, peeled, chopped
and seeded**
1 piece of orange peel (1 inch)
**1 can (20 ounces) unsweetened
crushed pineapple, undrained**

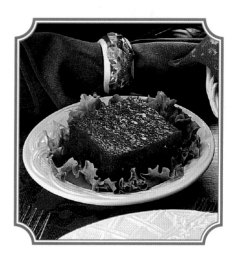

In a bowl, dissolve gelatin in water. Stir
in all remaining ingredients. Process in
small batches in a blender until coarsely
chopped. Pour into a 13-in. x 9-in. x 2-in.
dish or a 3-qt. serving bowl. Chill until set,
about 2-3 hours. **Yield:** 16 servings.

Exchanges: 1/2 Fruit

Nutritional Information

Serving Size: 1/16 recipe
Calories: 43
Sodium: 60 mg
Cholesterol: 0 mg

Carbohydrate: 9 gm
Protein: 1 gm
Fat: trace
Fiber: 2 gm

Minted Potato Salad

Shirley Glaab, Hattiesburg, Mississippi

In this unique potato salad, parsley adds a pretty green color while still allowing the subtle mint flavor to come through.

4 medium potatoes (1 pound)
1/2 cup chopped fresh parsley
3 tablespoons olive *or*
vegetable oil
2 tablespoons lemon juice
1 tablespoon chopped fresh mint
1 garlic clove, minced
1/2 teaspoon salt-free seasoning
blend
Pinch pepper

In a saucepan, cook potatoes in boiling water until tender. Peel and cube; place in a medium bowl. Combine remaining ingredients in a small bowl. Add to potatoes and mix well. Refrigerate for at least 1 hour before serving. **Yield:** 6 servings.

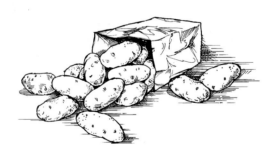

Exchanges: 1 Starch, 1 Fat
Nutritional Information

Serving Size: 1/2 cup
Calories: 130
Sodium: 4 mg
Cholesterol: 0 mg

Carbohydrate: 18 gm
Protein: 3 gm
Fat: 7 gm
Fiber: 2 gm

Sunflower Strawberry Salad

Betty Malone, Humboldt, Tennessee

We have an annual Strawberry Festival in our town, so recipes with strawberries are popular here. I've served this salad at luncheons and have always received a lot of compliments.

2 cups sliced fresh strawberries
1 medium apple, diced
1 cup seedless green grapes, halved
1/2 cup thinly sliced celery
1/4 cup raisins
1/2 cup strawberry light nonfat yogurt
2 tablespoons unsalted sunflower kernels
Lettuce leaves, optional

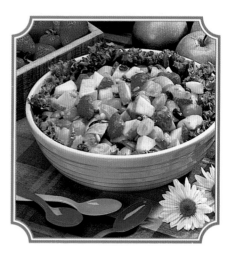

In a large bowl, combine strawberries, apple, grapes, celery and raisins. Stir in the yogurt. Cover and refrigerate for at least 1 hour. Just before serving, stir in sunflower kernels; toss. Serve on lettuce if desired. **Yield:** 6 servings.

Exchanges: 2 Fruit

Nutritional Information

Serving Size: 1/6 recipe
Calories: 102
Sodium: 21 mg
Cholesterol: 1 mg

Carbohydrate: 21 gm
Protein: 2 gm
Fat: 2 gm
Fiber: 3 gm

Spiral Pasta Salad

Darlene Kileel, Riverview, New Brunswick

I have two kids and am always on the go, so I appreciate recipes that I can make ahead of time. This dish is easy to fix and perfect for taking along on picnics.

3 cups cooked spiral pasta
1/2 cup chopped green pepper
1/2 cup sliced celery
1/2 cup chopped tomato
1/2 cup shredded carrot
DRESSING:
1/4 cup vegetable oil
1/4 cup cider vinegar
1/4 cup chopped onion
2 tablespoons ketchup
4 teaspoons sugar
1/2 teaspoon salt-free seasoning blend
1/4 teaspoon ground mustard
1/4 teaspoon paprika
1/4 teaspoon garlic powder
1/4 teaspoon dried oregano

In a large bowl, combine pasta, green pepper, celery, tomato and carrot. In a jar with tight-fitting lid, combine dressing ingredients; shake well. Pour over salad and toss. Chill. **Yield:** 8 servings.

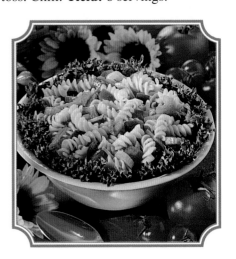

Exchanges: 1 Starch, 1 Fat, 1/2 Vegetable

Nutritional Information

Serving Size: 1/2 cup
Calories: 156
Sodium: 56 mg
Cholesterol: 0 mg

Carbohydrate: 21 gm
Protein: 3 gm
Fat: 7 gm
Fiber: 1 gm

Mixed Greens with Mushrooms

Sue Walker, Greentown, Indiana

This is a great year-round salad because you can use whatever greens are in season. The tarragon in the dressing is subtle but really adds to the flavor.

6 cups mixed salad greens
1 cup halved cherry tomatoes
1/2 pound fresh mushrooms, sliced
DRESSING:
  1 tablespoon cider *or* red
    wine vinegar
  1 tablespoon lemon juice
  1 tablespoon thinly sliced green
    onion
  1 tablespoon Dijon mustard

  1 tablespoon minced fresh parsley
  1/4 teaspoon salt-free seasoning
    blend
  1/4 teaspoon sugar
  1/8 teaspoon dried tarragon
Dash pepper

Toss greens, tomatoes and mushrooms in a large bowl. In a small bowl, whisk together dressing ingredients; pour over salad and serve immediately. **Yield:** 8 servings.

SELECTING SALAD GREENS. For the most nutrition, select the greenest lettuces you can find, such as romaine, spinach, endive, watercress and green and red leaf.

Exchanges: Free food

Nutritional Information

Serving Size: 1 cup
Calories: 22
Sodium: 61 mg
Cholesterol: 0 mg

Carbohydrate: 4 gm
Protein: 2 gm
Fat: trace
Fiber: 1 gm

Orange Buttermilk Salad

Lenore Wilson, Muskogee, Oklahoma

My family loves this salad, and I do, too, because it's so easy to make! The buttermilk adds a wonderful tang, making it a refreshing accompaniment to any meal.

1 can (20 ounces) unsweetened crushed pineapple, undrained
1 package (.6 ounce) sugar-free orange gelatin
2 cups buttermilk
1 carton (8 ounces) light frozen whipped topping, thawed

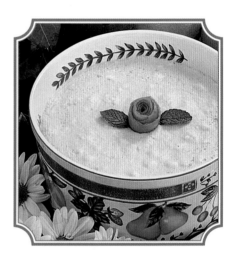

In a saucepan, bring pineapple with juice to a boil. Stir in the gelatin until dissolved. Remove from the heat; stir in buttermilk. Cool to room temperature. Fold in whipped topping. Pour into an 11-in. x 7-in. x 2-in. dish or 2-qt. bowl. Refrigerate for at least 4 hours. **Yield:** 10 servings.

Exchanges: 1/2 Fruit, 1/2 Skim Milk

Nutritional Information

Serving Size: 1/10 recipe
Calories: 101
Sodium: 96 mg
Cholesterol: 2 mg

Carbohydrate: 13 gm
Protein: 3 gm
Fat: 3 gm
Fiber: trace

Calico Tomato Salad

Donna Cline, Pensacola, Florida

This recipe has been in our family for years. We always appreciate this wonderful, eye-catching salad because it's so easy to prepare and delicious to eat.

5 medium tomatoes
1 small zucchini
1 small sweet yellow pepper
1/4 cup cider vinegar
2 tablespoons olive *or* vegetable oil
2 tablespoons minced fresh parsley
2 teaspoons sugar
1/4 teaspoon salt-free seasoning blend
1/2 teaspoon dried bail
1/4 teaspoon dried marjoram
1/8 teaspoon pepper

Cut tomatoes, zucchini and yellow pepper into 1/2-in. pieces; place in a large bowl. In a jar with tight-fitting lid, combine remaining ingredients; shake well. Pour over vegetables and toss. Serve immediately. **Yield:** 8 servings.

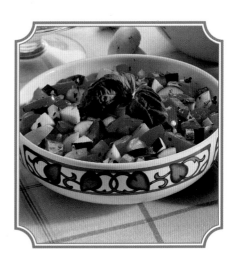

Exchanges: 1 Vegetable, 1/2 Fat

Nutritional Information

Serving Size: 3/4 cup
Calories: 56
Sodium: 8 mg
Cholesterol: 0 mg

Carbohydrate: 6 gm
Protein: 1 gm
Fat: 4 gm
Fiber: 1 gm

Apple Cottage Cheese Salad

Diane Sparrow, Osage, Iowa

*This refreshing salad is a welcome addition to any potluck or buffet.
I always receive recipe requests and come home with
an empty bowl...two great compliments for any cook!*

3 cups fat-free cottage cheese
2 small apples, chopped
1/4 cup raisins
2 teaspoons poppy seeds
2 tablespoons lemon juice
2 tablespoons honey
1/2 cup unsalted sunflower kernels

In a bowl, combine cottage cheese, apples, raisins and poppy seeds. Combine lemon juice and honey; add to apple mixture. Refrigerate. Just before serving, stir in sunflower kernels. **Yield:** 10 servings.

POPPY SEED POINTERS. To keep poppy seeds fresh, store them in an airtight container in the refrigerator for up to 6 months.

Exchanges: 1–1/2 Lean Meat, 1/2 Fruit

Nutritional Information

Serving Size: 1/2 cup
Calories: 131
Sodium: 224 mg
Cholesterol: 6 mg

Carbohydrate: 14 gm
Protein: 11 gm
Fat: 4 gm
Fiber: 2 gm

Garbanzo Cucumber Salad

Sharon Semph, Victorville, California

*This crisp, refreshing salad is great for a barbecue or potluck.
It can even be made ahead when you know your time is tight.*

1 can (15 ounces) **garbanzo beans,
   rinsed and drained**
1 medium **cucumber, sliced and
   quartered**
1/2 cup **sliced ripe olives**
1/3 cup **chopped red onion**
1/4 cup **minced fresh parsley**
  3 tablespoons **vegetable oil**
  3 tablespoons **cider** *or* **red
   wine vinegar**
  1 tablespoon **sugar**
  1 tablespoon **fresh lemon juice**
  2 **garlic cloves, minced**
1/2 teaspoon **grated lemon peel**
1/4 teaspoon **salt-free seasoning
  blend**
1/8 teaspoon **pepper**

In a medium bowl, combine beans, cucumber, olives, onion and parsley. In a jar with tight-fitting lid, combine remaining ingredients; shake well. Pour over vegetables and toss. Serve immediately or refrigerate for up to 24 hours. **Yield:** 8 servings.

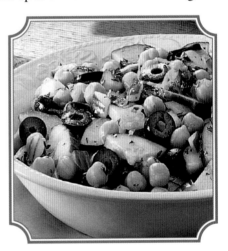

Exchanges: 1 Starch, 1 Fat
Nutritional Information

Serving Size: 1/2 cup
Calories: 132
Sodium: 234 mg
Cholesterol: 0 mg

Carbohydrate: 16 gm
Protein: 3 gm
Fat: 7 gm
Fiber: 3 gm

Mexican Potato Salad

Danette Hofer, Cedar Rapids, Iowa

This fun, fresh-tasting potato salad is a colorful and zesty variation of the average potato salad. It looks great and people love it.

1/4 cup low-sodium chicken broth
  2 tablespoons cider *or* white wine vinegar
  2 tablespoons pickled jalapeno pepper juice
  2 tablespoons olive *or* vegetable oil
1-1/2 pounds red potatoes
  1 cup sliced carrots
  2 celery ribs, thinly sliced
1/2 cup chopped onion
1/2 cup frozen peas, thawed
1/3 cup sliced green onions
  1 tablespoon minced pickled jalapeno peppers
1/4 teaspoon pepper

In a large bowl, combine the first four ingredients; set aside. Place potatoes in a saucepan and cover with water; bring to a boil. Cook until almost tender, about 15 minutes. Add carrots and cook until carrots and potatoes are tender; drain. When cool enough to handle, cube potatoes. Add potatoes and carrots to broth mixture. Add remaining ingredients; toss to coat. Serve at room temperature or slightly chilled. **Yield:** 12 servings.

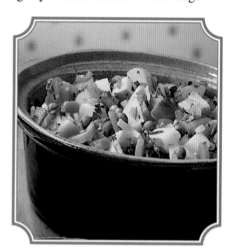

Exchanges: 1 Starch

Nutritional Information

Serving Size: 1/2 cup
Calories: 86
Sodium: 22 mg
Cholesterol: trace

Carbohydrate: 15 gm
Protein: 2 gm
Fat: 2 gm
Fiber: 2 gm

Green and Red Tomato Toss

Pauline Forrester, Titus, Alabama

Don't turn up your nose at green tomatoes. In this clever recipe, red and green tomatoes are topped with a savory oil and vinegar dressing.

1/2 cup olive *or* vegetable oil
3 tablespoons cider *or* red wine vinegar
2 tablespoons lemon juice
1 garlic clove, minced
1/2 teaspoon ground cumin
1/8 teaspoon pepper
3 medium red tomatoes, diced
3 medium green tomatoes, diced
1 medium red onion, thinly sliced into rings
3 tablespoons minced fresh basil *or* 1 tablespoon dried basil

In a small bowl or jar, combine oil, vinegar, lemon juice, garlic, cumin and pepper; mix well. Refrigerate. In a large salad bowl, combine the tomatoes, onion and basil. About 30 minutes before serving, add the dressing and toss. **Yield:** 14 servings.

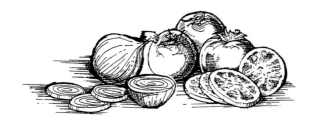

Exchanges: 1-1/2 Fat, 1/2 Vegetable

Nutritional Information

Serving Size: 1/14 recipe
Calories: 79
Sodium: 3 mg
Cholesterol: 0 mg

Carbohydrate: 3 gm
Protein: trace
Fat: 8 gm
Fiber: trace

Celebration Antipasto

Audrey Thibodeau, Mesa, Arizona

I made this marinated vegetable salad as part of a New Year's Eve buffet supper one year. It's a wonderful side dish for any gathering.

1 medium cucumber
1 medium zucchini, julienned
1 medium carrot, julienned
1 medium red onion, sliced
1 cup fresh broccoli florets
1 cup fresh cauliflowerets
1 can (2-1/4 ounces) sliced ripe
  olives, drained
1/2 cup olive *or* vegetable oil
1/4 cup cider *or* white wine vinegar
1 teaspoon dried oregano
1/2 teaspoon ground mustard
1/4 teaspoon garlic powder
1/4 teaspoon salt-free seasoning
  blend
1/8 teaspoon pepper
1/8 teaspoon celery salt

In a bowl, combine the vegetables and olives. In a small bowl, whisk oil, vinegar and seasonings. Pour over vegetables and toss. Refrigerate for 3 hours. Serve in a lettuce-lined bowl with a slotted spoon. **Yield:** 16 servings.

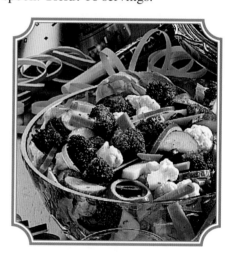

Exchanges: 1-1/2 Fat, 1/2 Vegetable
Nutritional Information

Serving Size: 1/16 recipe
Calories: 75
Sodium: 53 mg
Cholesterol: 0 mg

Carbohydrate: 3 gm
Protein: trace
Fat: 7 gm
Fiber: 1 gm

Green Bean Sesame Salad

Mildred Sherrer, Bay City, Texas

A friend brought this refreshing salad to a church luncheon and came prepared with copies of the recipe, saying someone always asks for it. I was sure to get a copy for myself.

1 pound fresh green beans
2 tablespoons olive *or* vegetable oil
1 tablespoon lemon juice
2 tablespoons sesame seeds, toasted
1 garlic clove, minced
1/2 teaspoon salt-free seasoning blend
1/2 teaspoon crushed red pepper flakes
1/8 teaspoon pepper

In a saucepan, cover beans with water; cook until crisp-tender. Drain and rinse in cold water; place in a serving bowl. Sprinkle with remaining ingredients; toss to coat. Serve at room temperature. **Yield:** 6 servings.

TOASTING SESAME SEEDS. You can toast sesame seeds either in a skillet over medium heat or in a 350° oven. Stir occasionally and toast only until golden brown.

Exchanges: 1 Vegetable, 1 Fat

Nutritional Information

Serving Size: 1/6 recipe
Calories: 82
Sodium: 5 mg
Cholesterol: 0 mg

Carbohydrate: 6 gm
Protein: 2 gm
Fat: 6 gm
Fiber: 1 gm

Dilly Pea Salad

Rita Applegate, La Mesa, California

This refreshing salad dresses up peas in a deliciously different way. I got the recipe from my best friend when I was just a young bride.

1 cup (8 ounces) nonfat sour cream
4 teaspoons lemon juice
4 teaspoons sliced green onion
2 teaspoons sugar
1 teaspoon dill weed
1/2 teaspoon curry powder
1/2 teaspoon salt-free seasoning blend
1/4 teaspoon pepper
2 packages (10 ounces *each*) frozen peas, thawed

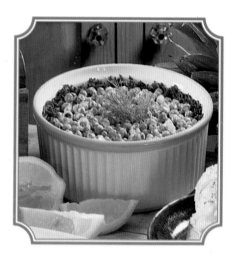

In a medium bowl, combine the first eight ingredients. Add peas; toss. Refrigerate until ready to serve. **Yield:** 6 servings.

Exchanges: 1 Starch, 1/2 Skim Milk

Nutritional Information

Serving Size: 1/6 recipe
Calories: 127
Sodium: 144 mg
Cholesterol: 3 mg

Carbohydrate: 23 gm
Protein: 8 gm
Fat: trace
Fiber: 5 gm

Peachy Applesauce Salad

Marcille Meyer, Battle Creek, Nebraska

I've been revising many recipes and creating new ones since my husband developed diabetes a couple of years ago. This makes a light side dish or dessert.

1 cup diet lemon-lime soda
1 package (.3 ounce) sugar-free
peach *or* mixed fruit gelatin
1 cup unsweetened applesauce
2 cups light whipped topping
1/8 teaspoon ground nutmeg
1/8 teaspoon vanilla extract
1 medium fresh peach, peeled
and chopped

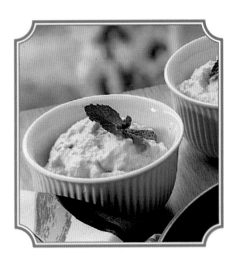

In a saucepan, bring soda to a boil. Remove from the heat; stir in gelatin until dissolved. Add applesauce; chill until partially set. Fold in whipped topping, nutmeg and vanilla. Fold in peach. Chill until firm. **Yield:** 6 servings.

Exchanges: 1 Fruit

Nutritional Information

Serving Size: 1/2 cup
Calories: 82
Sodium: trace
Cholesterol: 0 mg

Carbohydrate: 13 gm
Protein: trace
Fat: 3 gm
Fiber: 1 gm

Corn Slaw

Sue Burton, Frankfort, Kansas

My mother gave this recipe to me. It's one my husband and two daughters ask for often in summer, especially when we're having a grilled meal.

2 cups fresh *or* frozen corn, cooked and drained
1 cup diced carrots
1 cup diced green pepper
1/2 cup chopped onion
1/4 cup fat-free mayonnaise
1/4 cup nonfat sour cream
2 teaspoons vinegar
1 teaspoon prepared yellow mustard
1/4 teaspoon salt-free seasoning blend

In a salad bowl, toss corn, carrots, green pepper and onion. In a small bowl, combine remaining ingredients; pour over vegetables and mix well. Refrigerate for several hours before serving. **Yield:** 8 servings.

> **CUTTING KERNELS.** To cut kernels from corn-cobs, stand one end of the cob on a cutting board. Starting at the top, run a sharp knife down the cob, cutting deeply to remove whole kernels. One medium cob yields about 1/2 cup kernels.

Exchanges: 1 Vegetable, 1/2 Starch

Nutritional Information

Serving Size: 1/8 recipe
Calories: 69
Sodium: 73 mg
Cholesterol: trace

Carbohydrate: 2 gm
Protein: 2 gm
Fat: trace
Fiber: 2 gm

Sally's Potato Salad

Sally Burek, Fenton, Michigan

Broccoli, cauliflower, green beans and red pepper give traditional potato salad a new twist. It's a fresh-tasting dish that makes a nice addition to all your meals.

6 medium red potatoes, cubed
1-1/2 cups chopped celery
1-1/2 cups fresh broccoli florets
3/4 cup cut fresh green beans, blanched
1/2 cup fresh cauliflowerets
1/2 cup julienned sweet red pepper
1/4 cup fat-free Italian salad dressing
1/2 cup reduced-fat mayonnaise
2 teaspoons reduced-fat dry ranch salad dressing mix
1/4 teaspoon pepper

Cook potatoes in boiling water until tender; drain. In a large bowl, combine the potatoes, celery, broccoli, beans, cauliflower, red pepper and Italian dressing. Combine mayonnaise, salad dressing mix and pepper; pour over the vegetable mixture and toss to coat. Cover and refrigerate for at least 2 hours. **Yield:** 16 servings.

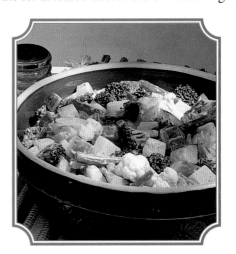

Exchanges: 1 Vegetable, 1/2 Starch

Nutritional Information

Serving Size: 1/2 cup
Calories: 74
Sodium: 105 mg
Cholesterol: trace

Carbohydrate: 12 gm
Protein: 2 gm
Fat: 3 gm
Fiber: 2 gm

Seven-Vegetable Medley

Kim Wiehe-Kaylor, Sidney, Ohio

*This fun, no-lettuce salad is popular at home or
when I take it to potlucks. It's colorful and crunchy!*

1-3/4 cups cauliflowerets
1-1/4 cups chopped cucumber
1 cup sliced celery
1/2 cup quartered cherry tomatoes
1/4 cup julienned green pepper
1/4 cup julienned sweet red pepper
2 tablespoons sliced green onions
1/4 cup fat-free salad dressing

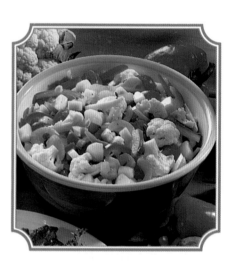

In a large bowl, combine all vegetables.
Pour dressing over; toss to coat. **Yield:** 5
servings.

Exchanges: 1 Vegetable
Nutritional Information

Serving Size: 1 cup
Calories: 27
Sodium: 35 mg
Cholesterol: 0 mg

Carbohydrate: 6 gm
Protein: 2 gm
Fat: trace
Fiber: 2 gm

Black 'n' White Bean Salad

Kay Ogden, Grants Pass, Oregon

*I created this cool, hearty side dish after tasting a
similar one in a restaurant. It goes together in no time
and complements most entrees.*

1 can (15 ounces) black beans,
    rinsed and drained
1 can (15 ounces) white kidney
    beans, rinsed and drained
1/2 cup chopped cucumber
1/2 cup chopped sweet red pepper
1/4 cup chopped onion
1/4 cup minced fresh cilantro *or*
    parsley
1/3 cup cider *or* red wine vinegar
1/4 cup olive *or* vegetable oil
1/2 teaspoon salt-free seasoning
    blend
1/4 teaspoon garlic powder
1/8 teaspoon pepper
Lettuce leaves, optional

In a large bowl, combine the first six ingredients. In a small bowl, whisk vinegar, oil and seasonings. Pour over bean
mixture and toss to coat. Cover and refrigerate until serving. Using a slotted
spoon, serve over lettuce if desired. **Yield:**
6 servings.

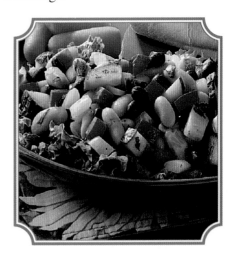

Exchanges: 1-1/2 Fat, 1 Starch, 1/2 Vegetable
Nutritional Information
Serving Size: 1/6 recipe
Calories: 205
Sodium: 367 mg
Cholesterol: 0 mg

Carbohydrate: 22 gm
Protein: 7 gm
Fat: 10 gm
Fiber: 7 gm

Apricot Aspic

Neva Jane Upp, Hutchinson, Kansas

*A family who usually passes up molded salads will
hunt for this fruity version at our covered-dish buffet.
Not only is it delicious, it adds color to any meal.*

2 cans (16 ounces *each***)
unsweetened apricot halves**
1/8 teaspoon salt
**1 package (.6 ounce) sugar-free
orange gelatin**
**1 can (6 ounces) unsweetened
frozen orange juice concentrate,
thawed**
1 tablespoon lemon juice
1 cup diet lemon-lime soda

Drain apricots, reserving 1-1/2 cups juice;
set apricots aside. In a small saucepan
over medium heat, bring apricot juice and
salt to a boil. Remove from the heat; add
gelatin and stir until dissolved. In a
blender, process apricots, orange juice
concentrate and lemon juice until smooth.
Add to gelatin mixture along with soda;
mix well. Pour into a 6-cup mold coated
with nonstick cooking spray. Refrigerate
until firm. **Yield:** 10 servings.

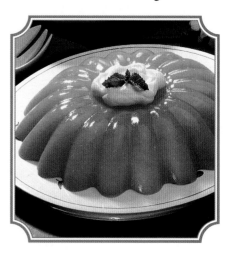

Exchanges: 1 Fruit
Nutritional Information

Serving Size: 1/10 recipe
Calories: 59
Sodium: 77 mg
Cholesterol: 0 mg

Carbohydrate: 12 gm
Protein: 2 gm
Fat: trace
Fiber: 2 gm

Broccoli Tomato Salad

Marie Hoyer, Hodgenville, Kentucky
(ALSO PICTURED ON FRONT COVER)

*Garden-fresh tomatoes and broccoli brighten this
salad with distinctive flavor and eye-catching color.*

**1 large bunch broccoli, separated
into florets
2 large tomatoes, cut into wedges
3/4 cup sliced fresh mushrooms
2 green onions, sliced
DRESSING:**
   **1/2 cup olive *or* vegetable oil
1/3 cup cider *or* tarragon vinegar
2 tablespoons water
1 teaspoon lemon juice
1 teaspoon sugar
1 teaspoon salt-free seasoning
blend
3/4 teaspoon dried thyme
1 garlic clove, minced
1/2 teaspoon celery seed
1/4 teaspoon Italian seasoning
1/4 teaspoon salt-free lemon-pepper
seasoning
1/4 teaspoon paprika
1/4 teaspoon ground mustard**

Cook broccoli in a small amount of water for 5 minutes or until crisp-tender.

Rinse with cold water and drain. Place in a large bowl; add tomatoes, mushrooms and onions. Combine dressing ingredients in a jar with a tight-fitting lid; shake well. Pour over salad; toss gently. Cover and refrigerate for 1 hour. Serve with a slotted spoon. **Yield**: 8 servings.

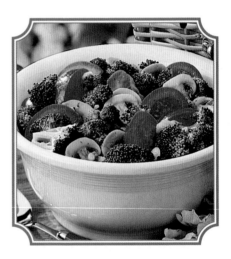

Exchanges: 2-1/2 Fat, 1-1/2 Vegetable

Nutritional Information

Serving Size: 1/8 recipe
Calories: 155
Sodium: 22 mg
Cholesterol: 0 mg

Carbohydrate: 8 gm
Protein: 3 gm
Fat: 14 gm
Fiber: 3 gm

Wild Rice Salad

Lyn Graebert, Park Falls, Wisconsin

I first tried this recipe at a luncheon during a holiday home tour. Since cranberries grow well in this area, I love to use the dried variety to give recipes like this hearty salad color and tang.

4 cups cooked wild rice (without added salt)
1 can (8 ounces) sliced water chestnuts, drained and chopped
1/2 cup thinly sliced celery
1/2 cup chopped green pepper
1/2 cup frozen peas, thawed
1/2 cup dried cranberries
1/4 cup thinly sliced green onions
1/4 cup minced fresh parsley
1/3 cup cranberry juice
1/3 cup vinegar
2 teaspoons olive *or* vegetable oil
3/4 teaspoon dried basil
3/4 teaspoon sugar
3/4 teaspoon salt-free seasoning blend
1/4 teaspoon pepper
1/2 cup chopped pecans

In a large bowl, combine the first eight ingredients. In a small bowl, combine cranberry juice, vinegar, oil, basil, sugar, seasoning blend and pepper; mix well. Pour over rice mixture and toss to coat. Refrigerate overnight. Just before serving, stir in pecans. **Yield:** 12 servings.

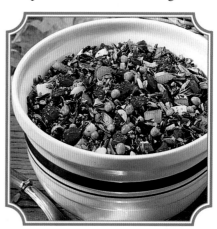

Exchanges: 1 Vegetable, 1 Starch, 1/2 Fat

Nutritional Information

Serving Size: 1/2 cup
Calories: 134
Sodium: 16 mg
Cholesterol: 0 mg
Carbohydrate: 22 gm
Protein: 3 gm
Fat: 4 gm
Fiber: 3 gm

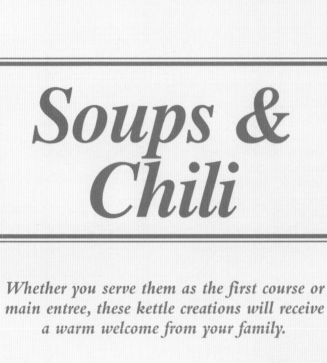

Soups & Chili

Whether you serve them as the first course or main entree, these kettle creations will receive a warm welcome from your family.

Slow-Cooked Chili

Sue Call, Beech Grove, Indiana

*This hearty chili can cook for up to 10 hours on low.
It's so good to come home to after a long day away.*

2 pounds lean ground beef
**2 cans (16 ounces *each*) kidney
 beans, rinsed and drained**
**2 cans (14-1/2 ounces *each*)
 no-salt-added tomatoes,
 undrained and cut up**
**1 can (8 ounces) no-salt-added
 tomato sauce**
2 medium onions, chopped
1 medium green pepper, chopped
2 garlic cloves, minced
2 tablespoons chili powder
**2 teaspoons salt-free seasoning
 blend**
1 teaspoon pepper
**1 cup shredded fat-free cheddar
 cheese**

In a skillet, brown beef; drain. Transfer to a slow cooker. Add the next nine ingredients. Cover and cook on low for 8-10 hours or on high for 4 hours. Garnish individual servings with cheese. **Yield:** 10 servings.

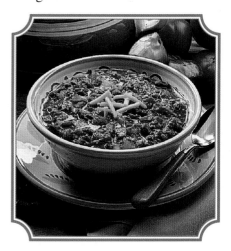

Exchanges: 3 Lean Meat, 1-1/2 Starch, 1-1/2 Vegetable

Nutritional Information

Serving Size: 1 cup
Calories: 316
Sodium: 175 mg
Cholesterol: 34 mg

Carbohydrate: 29 gm
Protein: 30 gm
Fat: 9 gm
Fiber: 10 gm

Creamy Onion Soup

Naomi Giddis, Two Buttes, Colorado

My husband, Dale, works at a grain elevator and is outside in all kinds of weather. He always appreciates warming up with a bowl of this soup.

1 pound yellow onions (about 3 medium), sliced
2 tablespoons margarine
4 cups low-sodium chicken broth
Dash *each* **pepper and dried thyme**
1/4 teaspoon salt-free seasoning blend
2 cups skim milk, *divided*
1/3 cup all-purpose flour

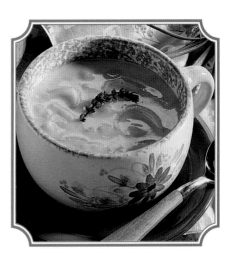

In a 3-qt. saucepan over medium heat, saute onions in margarine. Add broth, pepper, thyme and seasoning blend; bring to a boil. Reduce heat; cover and simmer for 20 minutes. Add 1-2/3 cups milk. Stir flour into remaining milk until smooth; add to soup. Bring to a boil; boil and stir for 2 minutes or until thickened. **Yield:** 6 servings (1-1/2 quarts).

Exchanges: 1-1/2 Vegetable, 1/2 Starch, 1/2 Skim Milk, 1/2 Fat

Nutritional Information

Serving Size: 1 cup
Calories: 135
Sodium: 154 mg
Cholesterol: 4 mg

Carbohydrate: 17 gm
Protein: 7 gm
Fat: 5 gm
Fiber: 2 gm

Hungarian Goulash Soup

Julie Polakowski, West Allis, Wisconsin

This soup, similar to one my mother made years ago, is brimming with vegetables.

1-1/4 pounds beef stew meat, cut
    into 1-inch cubes
  2 tablespoons olive *or* vegetable
    oil, *divided*
  4 medium onions, chopped
  6 garlic cloves, minced
  2 teaspoons paprika
1/2 teaspoon caraway seeds, crushed
1/2 teaspoon pepper
1/4 teaspoon cayenne pepper
  1 teaspoon salt-free seasoning blend
  2 cans (14-1/2 ounces *each*) low-
    sodium beef broth
  2 cups cubed peeled potatoes
  2 cups sliced carrots
  2 cups cubed peeled rutabagas
  2 cans (28 ounces *each*) diced
    tomatoes, undrained
  1 large sweet red pepper, chopped
  1 cup (8 ounces) nonfat sour cream

In a Dutch oven over medium heat, brown beef in 1 tablespoon oil. Remove beef; drain drippings. Heat remaining oil in the same pan; saute onions and garlic for 8-10 minutes over medium heat or until lightly browned. Add paprika, caraway, pepper, cayenne and seasoning blend; cook and stir for 1 minute. Return beef to pan. Add broth, potatoes, carrots and rutabagas; bring to a boil. Reduce heat; cover and simmer for 1-1/2 hours. Add tomatoes and red pepper; return to a boil. Reduce heat; cover and simmer 30-40 minutes longer or until meat and vegetables are tender. Serve with sour cream. **Yield:** 15 servings.

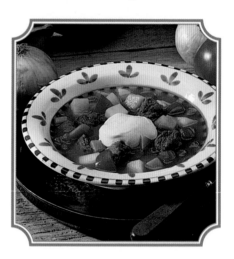

Exchanges: 2 Lean Meat, 2 Vegetable, 1/2 Fat

Nutritional Information

Serving Size: 1 cup
Calories: 207
Sodium: 376 mg
Cholesterol: 40 mg

Carbohydrate: 20 gm
Protein: 16 gm
Fat: 7 gm
Fiber: 3 gm

Carrot Leek Soup

Norma Meyers, Huntsville, Arkansas

*The vegetables in this pretty golden soup are pureed,
so you can disguise them from picky eaters!
Filled with vitamins, this is a filling meal in inself.*

1 medium leek, thinly sliced
4 teaspoons reduced-fat
   margarine
6 medium carrots, sliced
2 medium potatoes, peeled and
   cubed
3 cans (14-1/2 ounces *each*)
   low-sodium chicken broth
2 cups skim milk
1/8 teaspoon pepper

In a large saucepan, saute leek in margarine until tender. Add carrots, potatoes and broth; bring to a boil. Reduce heat; cover and simmer until vegetables are tender. Cool to room temperature. Remove vegetables with a slotted spoon to a blender or food processor. Add enough cooking liquid to cover; blend until smooth. Return to pan. Stir in milk and pepper; heat through. **Yield:** 10 servings.

LOOK FOR LEEKS with crisp, bright green leaves and unblemished white portions. Before using, trim the root end and remove the upper green leaves. If leeks are to be sliced, cut the leek open lengthwise down one side and rinse under cold running water, separating the leaves.

Exchanges: 1 Vegetable, 1/2 Starch
Nutritional Information
Serving Size: 1 cup
Calories: 82
Sodium: 101 mg
Cholesterol: 2 mg

Carbohydrate: 14 gm
Protein: 4 gm
Fat: 1 gm
Fiber: 2 gm

Pasta and Lentil Soup

Marie Herr, Berea, Ohio

This is a great soup to share with friends who are under the weather. I also like to layer the dry ingredients in a pretty jar, attach the recipe and give it as a gift.

3-1/2 cups water
1/2 cup uncooked small pasta
  (shells, elbow macaroni, etc.)
1/4 cup dry lentils
2 tablespoons grated Parmesan
  cheese
1 tablespoon dried minced onion
1 tablespoon low-sodium chicken
  bouillon granules

1-1/2 teaspoons dried vegetable flakes
1 teaspoon dried parsley flakes
1/2 teaspoon dried oregano
1/8 teaspoon garlic powder

Combine all ingredients in a 2-qt. saucepan; bring to a boil over medium heat. Reduce heat; cover and simmer for 25-30 minutes or until pasta and lentils are tender. **Yield:** 4 servings.

A LESSON IN LENTILS. Choose plump-looking dry lentils and discard any that are shriveled or spotted. Tightly wrap dry lentils, store in a cool, dry place and use within a year.

Exchanges: 1 Starch, 1/2 Lean Meat

Nutritional Information

Serving Size: 1 cup
Calories: 102
Sodium: 62 mg
Cholesterol: 3 mg

Carbohydrate: 16 gm
Protein: 7 gm
Fat: 1 gm
Fiber: 4 gm

Confetti Bean Chili

Kathleen Drott, Pineville, Louisiana

*A medley of vegetables and beans adds
color and appeal to this recipe. It's a tasty way to
get more vegetables into your diet.*

1 large onion, chopped
2 cans (14-1/2 ounces *each*)
  low-sodium chicken broth
2 garlic cloves, minced
3 tablespoons chili powder
1-1/2 teaspoons ground cumin
1/2 teaspoon dried oregano
1 pound carrots, sliced
1 pound red potatoes, cubed
2 cans (14-1/2 ounces *each*)
  no-salt-added tomatoes,
  undrained and cut up *or* 3 cups
  diced fresh tomatoes
1 can (16 ounces) kidney
  beans, rinsed and drained
1 can (15 ounces) black beans,
  rinsed and drained
1 can (15 ounces) garbanzo
  beans, rinsed and drained
2-1/2 cups water

In a Dutch oven, simmer onion in broth for 5 minutes. Add next six ingredients; bring to a boil. Reduce heat. Cover; simmer 10 minutes. Add remaining ingredients. Cover; simmer 20 minutes. **Yield:** 12 servings.

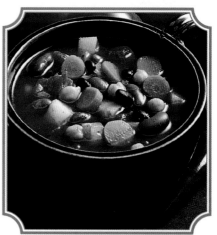

Exchanges: 2 Vegetable, 1–1/2 Starch
Nutritional Information

Serving Size: 1 cup
Calories: 201
Sodium: 279 mg
Cholesterol: 1 mg

Carbohydrate: 39 gm
Protein: 10 gm
Fat: 2 gm
Fiber: 10 gm

Harvest Squash Soup

Mrs. H.L. Sosnowski, Grand Island, New York

This soup is perfect for a group after an autumn outing. The combination of squash, applesauce and spices gives it an appealing flavor.

1-1/2 cups chopped onion
  1 tablespoon vegetable oil
  4 cups mashed cooked
    butternut squash
  3 cups low-sodium chicken broth
  2 cups unsweetened applesauce
1-1/2 cups skim milk
  1 bay leaf
  1 tablespoon lime juice
  1 tablespoon sugar
  1 teaspoon curry powder
  1/2 teaspoon ground cinnamon
  1/2 teaspoon salt-free seasoning
    blend
  1/4 teaspoon pepper
  1/4 teaspoon ground nutmeg

In a large saucepan or Dutch oven, saute onion in oil until tender. Add the remaining ingredients; simmer, uncovered, for 30 minutes. Discard bay leaf. **Yield:** 10 servings (2-1/2 quarts).

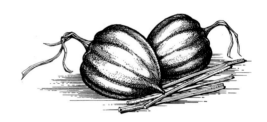

Exchanges: 1-1/2 Vegetable, 1/2 Fruit, 1/2 Fat

Nutritional Information

Serving Size: 1 cup
Calories: 100
Sodium: 56 mg
Cholesterol: 2 mg

Carbohydrate: 19 gm
Protein: 3 gm
Fat: 2 gm
Fiber: 3 gm

Mushroom Barley Soup

Lynn Thomas, London, Ontario

A friend at work shared the recipe for this wonderful soup. With beef, barley and vegetables, it's hearty enough to be a meal. A big steaming bowl is so satisfying on a cold day.

1-1/2 pounds boneless beef chuck, trimmed and cut into 3/4-inch cubes
1 tablespoon vegetable oil
2 cups finely chopped onion
1 cup diced carrots
1/2 cup sliced celery
1 pound fresh mushrooms, sliced
2 garlic cloves, minced
1/2 teaspoon dried thyme
1 can (14-1/2 ounces) low-sodium beef broth
1 can (14-1/2 ounces) low-sodium chicken broth
2 cups water
1/2 cup medium pearl barley
1 teaspoon salt-free seasoning blend
1/2 teaspoon pepper
3 tablespoons chopped fresh parsley

In a Dutch oven or soup kettle, brown meat in oil. Remove meat with a slotted spoon and set aside. Saute onion, carrots and celery in drippings over medium heat until tender, about 5 minutes. Add mushrooms, garlic and thyme; cook and stir for 3 minutes. Add broths, water, barley, seasoning blend and pepper. Return meat to pan; bring to a boil. Reduce heat; cover and simmer for 1-1/2 to 2 hours or until barley and meat are tender. Add parsley. **Yield:** 11 servings (2-3/4 quarts).

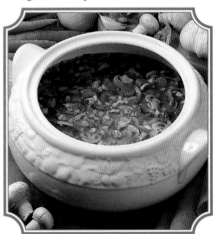

Exchanges: 1-1/2 Lean Meat, 1-1/2 Vegetable, 1 Starch, 1/2 Fat

Nutritional Information

Serving Size: 1 cup
Calories: 229
Sodium: 69 mg
Cholesterol: 38 mg

Carbohydrate: 22 gm
Protein: 16 gm
Fat: 9 gm
Fiber: 4 gm

Slow-Cooker Vegetable Soup

Heather Thurmeier, Pense, Saskatchewan

What a treat to come home from work and have this savory soup ready to eat. It's a nice traditional beef soup with old-fashioned goodness.

1 pound boneless round steak, cut into 1/2-inch cubes
1 can (14-1/2 ounces) no-salt-added tomatoes, undrained and cut up
3 cups water
2 medium potatoes, peeled and cubed
2 medium onions, diced
3 celery ribs, sliced
2 carrots, sliced
3 low-sodium beef bouillon cubes
1/2 teaspoon dried basil
1/2 teaspoon dried oregano
1/2 teaspoon salt-free seasoning blend
1/4 teaspoon pepper
1-1/2 cups frozen mixed vegetables

In a slow cooker, combine the first 12 ingredients. Cover and cook on high for 6 hours. Add vegetables; cover and cook on high 2 hours longer or until the meat and vegetables are tender. **Yield:** 8 servings (about 2-1/2 quarts).

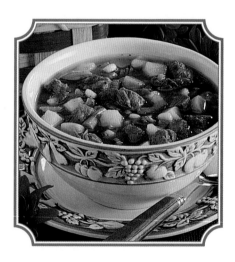

Exchanges: 2 Lean Meat, 1 Vegetable, 1/2 Starch

Nutritional Information

Serving Size: 1 cup
Calories: 183
Sodium: 102 mg
Cholesterol: 48 mg

Carbohydrate: 16 gm
Protein: 23 gm
Fat: 3 gm
Fiber: 4 gm

Chicken Chili

Lisa Goodman, Bloomington, Minnesota

Loaded with hearty beans and chicken, this
zippy chili really warms us up on chilly winter nights.

4-1/2 cups low-sodium chicken broth
  2 cans (15 ounces *each*) black
    beans, rinsed and drained
  1/2 cup *each* chopped green, sweet
    yellow and red pepper
  1/4 cup chopped onion
  1 tablespoon chili powder
1-1/2 teaspoons paprika
  1 to 1-1/2 teaspoons pepper
  1 to 1-1/2 teaspoons crushed red
    pepper flakes
  1 to 1-1/2 teaspoons ground
    cumin
  1/2 teaspoon salt-free seasoning
    blend
Dash cayenne pepper
  2 cups cubed cooked chicken
    breast

In a 3-qt. saucepan, bring broth to a boil. Reduce heat; add beans, peppers, onion and seasonings. Cover and simmer 15 minutes. Add chicken; simmer for 30 minutes. **Yield:** 7 servings.

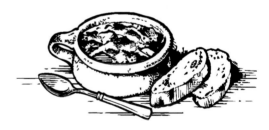

Exchanges: 2 Lean Meat, 1 Starch, 1/2 Vegetable

Nutritional Information

Serving Size: 1 cup
Calories: 201
Sodium: 474 mg
Cholesterol: 36 mg

Carbohydrate: 20 gm
Protein: 21 gm
Fat: 3 gm
Fiber: 7 gm

Canadian Cheese Soup

Jolene Roudebush, Troy, Michigan

*My family loves Canadian bacon, but I don't run across
a lot of dishes that call for this pork product. Everyone was thrilled
the first time I offered this succulent soup.*

3 cups low-sodium chicken broth
4 medium potatoes, peeled and
   diced
2 celery ribs, diced
1 medium carrot, diced
1 small onion, diced
6 ounces Canadian bacon, trimmed
   and diced
2 tablespoons margarine
2 tablespoons all-purpose flour
1 cup skim milk
2 cups (8 ounces) shredded
   reduced-fat cheddar cheese
1/8 teaspoon pepper

In a Dutch oven or soup kettle, combine the first five ingredients; bring to a boil. Reduce heat; cover and simmer for 20 minutes or until vegetables are very tender. With a potato masher, mash vegetables several times. Add bacon; continue to simmer. Meanwhile, melt margarine in a small saucepan; stir in the flour and cook, stirring constantly, for 1 minute. Gradually whisk in milk. Bring to a boil; boil and stir for 2 minutes (mixture will be thick). Add to vegetable mixture, stirring constantly. Remove from the heat; add cheese and pepper. Stir just until cheese is melted. **Yield:** 8 servings (2 quarts).

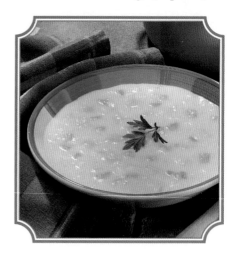

Exchanges: 1 Lean Meat, 1 Starch, 1 Fat, 1/2 Vegetable

Nutritional Information

Serving Size: 1 cup
Calories: 198
Sodium: 571 mg
Cholesterol: 19 mg

Carbohydrate: 21 gm
Protein: 16 gm
Fat: 7 gm
Fiber: 2 gm

Black Bean Soup

Audrey Thibodeau, Mesa, Arizona

Here's an economical meal that doesn't skimp on flavor. Hearty black beans make up for the meat, and the peppers add just the right splash of color.

1 pound dry black beans
1-1/2 quarts low-sodium chicken broth
1 quart water
1-1/2 cups chopped onions
1 cup thinly sliced celery
1 large carrot, chopped
1/2 cup *each* chopped green, sweet yellow and red peppers
2 garlic cloves, minced
3 tablespoons olive *or* vegetable oil
1/4 cup no-salt-added tomato paste
3 tablespoons minced fresh parsley
1 tablespoon chopped fresh oregano *or* 1 teaspoon dried oregano
1 tablespoon chopped fresh thyme *or* 1 teaspoon dried thyme
1-1/2 teaspoons ground cumin
1 teaspoon pepper
3/4 teaspoon salt-free seasoning blend
3 bay leaves

In a Dutch oven or soup kettle, combine beans, broth and water; bring to a boil. Reduce heat; cover and simmer for 1-1/2 hours or until beans are tender. Meanwhile, in a large skillet, saute onions, celery, carrot, peppers and garlic in oil until tender. Add the next seven ingredients; mix well. Add to beans along with bay leaves; bring to a boil. Reduce heat; cover and simmer for 1 hour. Discard bay leaves. **Yield:** 12 servings (3 quarts).

Exchanges: 1-1/2 Starch, 1-1/2 Vegetable, 1/2 Fat
Nutritional Information
Serving Size: 1 cup
Calories: 203
Sodium: 77 mg
Cholesterol: 2 mg
Carbohydrate: 31 gm
Protein: 10 gm
Fat: 4 gm
Fiber: 5 gm

Vegetable Chili

Charlene Martorana, Madison, Ohio

This chili, packed with beans and vegetables, has an appealing red color and fabulous flavor. I always make a large batch so that everyone can have seconds.

2 large onions, chopped
1 medium green pepper, chopped
3 garlic cloves, minced
1 tablespoon vegetable oil
1/2 cup water
2 medium carrots, cut into chunks
2 medium potatoes, peeled and cubed
1 can (14-1/2 ounces) low-sodium chicken broth
1 to 2 tablespoons chili powder
2 tablespoons sugar
1 teaspoon ground cumin
3/4 teaspoon dried oregano
1 small zucchini, sliced 1/4 inch thick
1 small yellow squash, sliced 1/4 inch thick
2 cans (28 ounces *each*) crushed tomatoes
1/3 cup ketchup
1 can (16 ounces) kidney beans, rinsed and drained
1 can (15 ounces) garbanzo beans, rinsed and drained
1 can (15 ounces) black beans, rinsed and drained
1 can (15-1/2 ounces) black-eyed peas, rinsed and drained

In a Dutch oven or soup kettle, saute onions, green pepper and garlic in oil until tender. Add water and carrots; cover and cook over medium-low heat for 5 minutes. Add potatoes, broth, chili powder, sugar, cumin and oregano; cover and cook for 10 minutes. Add zucchini, squash, tomatoes and ketchup; bring to a boil. Reduce heat; cover and simmer for 15 minutes. Stir in beans and peas; simmer for 10 minutes. **Yield:** 12 servings.

Exchanges: 1-1/2 Vegetable, 1 Starch
Nutritional Information
Serving Size: 1/12 recipe
Calories: 116
Sodium: 284 mg
Cholesterol: 1 mg

Carbohydrate: 24 gm
Protein: 4 gm
Fat: 2 gm
Fiber: 4 gm

Golden Autumn Soup

Janet Willick, St. Michael, Alberta

*Here's a great way to use the freshest produce harvested
in fall. It's a hot and hearty soup you can
make for everyday dinners and special-occasion suppers.*

**5 medium parsnips, peeled and
   chopped**
5 medium carrots, sliced
2 medium onions, chopped
**1 medium sweet potato, peeled and
   chopped**
**1 medium turnip, peeled and
   chopped**
2 celery ribs, sliced
2 bay leaves
**3 cans (14-1/2 ounces *each*) low-
   sodium chicken broth**
2 cups evaporated skim milk
1 teaspoon dried tarragon
1/4 teaspoon pepper

In a soup kettle or Dutch oven, combine the first eight ingredients; simmer for 30 minutes or until vegetables are tender. Discard bay leaves. Cool for 20 minutes. Puree in small batches in a blender; return to kettle. Add milk, tarragon and pepper; heat through. **Yield:** 12 servings (3 quarts).

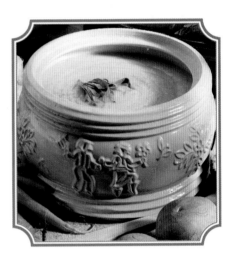

Exchanges: 1 Starch, 1 Vegetable, 1/2 Skim Milk

Nutritional Information

Serving Size: 1 cup
Calories: 145
Sodium: 149 mg
Cholesterol: 4 mg

Carbohydrate: 28 gm
Protein: 7 gm
Fat: 1 gm
Fiber: 5 gm

Lemon Asparagus Soup

Darlene Swille, Green Bay, Wisconsin

We have a small asparagus patch, and my husband and I wait eagerly for this tasty vegetable to appear every spring. We're pleased to use our precious harvest in this soup. Lemon and nutmeg give it a surprising spark.

1 medium onion, chopped
1/2 cup chopped celery
1/4 cup reduced-fat margarine
2 tablespoons cornstarch
1 cup water
2 low-sodium chicken
   bouillon cubes
3/4 pound fresh asparagus,
   trimmed and cut into 1-inch
   pieces
2 cups skim milk
1/4 to 1/2 teaspoon grated lemon
   peel
1/8 teaspoon ground nutmeg
1/8 teaspoon salt-free seasoning blend

In a 2-qt. saucepan, saute the onion and celery in margarine until tender. Dissolve cornstarch in water; add to the saucepan with bouillon. Bring to a boil over medium heat; cook and stir for 2 minutes. Add asparagus. Reduce heat; cover and simmer until asparagus is crisp-tender, about 3-4 minutes. Stir in the milk, lemon peel, nutmeg and seasoning blend. Cover and simmer for 25 minutes, stirring occasionally. **Yield:** 4 servings.

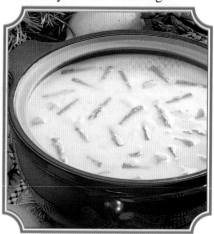

Exchanges: 2 Fat, 1-1/2 Vegetable, 1/2 Starch

Nutritional Information

Serving Size: 1 cup
Calories: 172
Sodium: 265 mg
Cholesterol: 4 mg

Carbohydrate: 18 gm
Protein: 9 gm
Fat: 8 gm
Fiber: 2 gm

Curried Pumpkin Soup

Eleanor Dunbar, Peoria, Illinois

This soup is wonderfully warming on an autumn day.
The subtle curry flavor enhances the pumpkin.

1 small onion, chopped
1 teaspoon vegetable oil
2 cups low-sodium chicken broth
1-1/2 cups cooked *or* canned pumpkin
1 tablespoon lemon juice
1 teaspoon curry powder
1 teaspoon sugar
1/2 teaspoon salt-free seasoning
   blend
Dash pepper
1/2 cup evaporated skim milk
Chopped fresh parsley

In a saucepan over medium heat, saute the onion in oil until tender. Add broth, pumpkin, lemon juice, curry powder, sugar, seasoning blend and pepper; bring to a boil. Reduce heat; cover and simmer for 15 minutes. Stir in milk; heat through. Garnish with parsley. **Yield:** 4 servings.

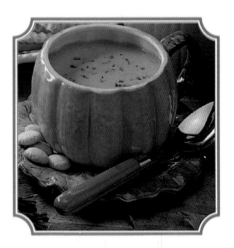

Exchanges: 1 Starch, 1/2 Vegetable

Nutritional Information

Serving Size: 1 cup
Calories: 98
Sodium: 611 mg
Cholesterol: 2 mg

Carbohydrate: 16 gm
Protein: 5 gm
Fat: 2 gm
Fiber: 3 gm

Surprise Clam Chowder

Evelyn Whalin, Denver, Colorado

When family and friends first sampled this stew over 40 years ago, they were pleasantly surprised by the combination of ingredients. Now my family requests it often.

1 can (14-1/2 ounces) no-salt-added tomatoes, undrained and cut up
1 cup water
1/2 cup diced peeled potato
1/4 cup diced green pepper
1/4 cup diced onion
1/4 teaspoon garlic powder
1/4 teaspoon chili powder
1 cup diced fully cooked low-sodium ham
1 can (7-1/2 ounces) minced clams, undrained

In a saucepan, combine the first seven ingredients. Cover and simmer for 25-30 minutes or until vegetables are tender. Add ham and clams; heat through. **Yield:** 4 servings.

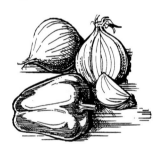

Exchanges: 2 Lean Meat, 1-1/2 Vegetable

Nutritional Information

Serving Size: 1 cup
Calories: 150
Sodium: 783 mg
Cholesterol: 39 mg

Carbohydrate: 13 gm
Protein: 17 gm
Fat: 3 gm
Fiber: 2 gm

Mom's Special Chicken Soup

Cookie Curci-Wright, San Jose, California

Nothing is more comforting than this chicken soup. A single bowl can soothe anything from the common cold to a stressful day.

1 broiler/fryer chicken (3-1/2
   pounds), skin removed
3 quarts water
1 medium onion, quartered
4 celery ribs
2 low-sodium chicken bouillon
   cubes
2 parsley sprigs
1 garlic clove
2-1/2 teaspoons salt-free seasoning
   blend
  1/2 cup thinly sliced carrots
  1/2 cup chopped fresh parsley
   3 cups cooked rice

Place chicken and water in a large kettle or Dutch oven; bring to a boil. Reduce heat; add onion, celery, bouillon, parsley sprigs, garlic and seasoning blend. Cover and simmer until the chicken is tender, about 1 hour. Remove chicken; allow to cool. Strain and reserve broth; discard vegeta-bles. Add carrots to broth and simmer until tender, about 15 minutes. Debone chicken; cut into cubes. Add chicken and chopped parsley to broth; heat through. Ladle into bowls; add rice to each bowl. **Yield:** 14 servings (3-1/2 quarts).

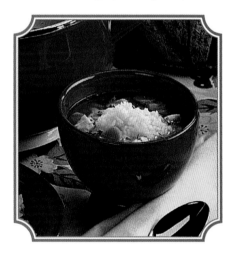

Exchanges: 2 Lean Meat, 1 Fat, 1/2 Vegetable, 1/2 Starch

Nutritional Information

Serving Size: 1 cup
Calories: 197
Sodium: 74 mg
Cholesterol: 49 mg

Carbohydrate: 12 gm
Protein: 14 gm
Fat: 10 gm
Fiber: 1 gm

Winter Vegetable Soup

Mavis Diment, Marcus, Iowa

I've enjoyed this for years because it tastes good, is simple to make and doesn't leave a lot of leftovers. When there's a chill in the air, a steaming bowl of this savory soup is welcome.

1/2 cup sliced green onions
1 tablespoon vegetable oil
1 can (14-1/2 ounces) low-sodium chicken broth
1 small potato, peeled and cubed
1 large carrot, sliced
1/4 teaspoon dried thyme
1 cup broccoli florets
1/4 teaspoon salt-free seasoning blend
1/8 teaspoon pepper

In a medium saucepan, saute onions in oil until tender. Add the next four ingredients; bring to a boil. Reduce heat; simmer, uncovered, for 5 minutes. Add the broccoli, seasoning blend and pepper; simmer, uncovered, for 7 minutes or until vegetables are tender. **Yield:** 2 servings.

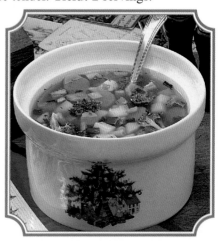

Exchanges: 1-1/2 Vegetable, 1 Starch, 1 Fat, 1/2 Lean Meat

Nutritional Information

Serving Size: 1/2 recipe
Calories: 184
Sodium: 154 mg
Cholesterol: 4 mg

Carbohydrate: 23 gm
Protein: 7 gm
Fat: 9 gm
Fiber: 4 gm

Beans and Barley Chili

Gail Applegate, Myrtle Beach, South Carolina

Most folks have heard of barley soup, but this barley chili takes them by surprise. My variation features a delectable combination of beans and seasonings.

1 cup medium pearl barley
2 cups chopped onion
2 cups chopped sweet
 red pepper
1 tablespoon vegetable oil
1 tablespoon minced garlic
2 tablespoons chili powder
1-1/2 teaspoons ground cumin
1/8 teaspoon cayenne pepper
1 can (16 ounces) kidney
 beans, rinsed and drained
1 can (15-1/2 ounces) black-
 eyed peas, rinsed and drained

1 can (15 ounces) black beans,
 rinsed and drained
1 can (14-1/2 ounces) reduced-
 sodium fat-free chicken broth
1 can (14-1/2 ounces) no-salt-
 added stewed tomatoes

Cook barley without adding salt; drain. Saute onion and red pepper in oil for 5 minutes. Add barley and remaining ingredients; bring to a boil. Reduce heat; simmer 20 minutes. **Yield:** 12 servings.

PEARL BARLEY has the outer shell removed and has been polished or "pearled". Store in an airtight container in a cool, dry place for 1 year.

Exchanges: 2 Starch, 2 Vegetable

Nutritional Information

Serving Size: 1 cup
Calories: 209
Sodium: 242 mg
Cholesterol: 1 mg

Carbohydrate: 38 gm
Protein: 10 gm
Fat: 2 gm
Fiber: 10 gm

Cabbage Soup

Terry Dunn, Kenai, Alaska

Folks are sure to comment on the great blend of spices and the hearty addition of cabbage in this soup.

1 pound ground turkey breast
1 large onion, chopped
4 large potatoes, peeled and cubed
4 large carrots, grated
4 celery ribs, chopped
1/2 small head cabbage, shredded
1/4 cup uncooked long grain rice
1 quart water
2 cans (14-1/2 ounces *each*) no-salt-added tomatoes, undrained and cut up
1 can (8 ounces) tomato sauce
1 can (16 ounces) kidney beans, rinsed and drained
2 bay leaves
1 teaspoon dried basil
1 teaspoon dried thyme
3/4 teaspoon pepper
1/2 teaspoon dill weed
1 teaspoon salt-free seasoning blend

In a Dutch oven or soup kettle, brown meat and onion; drain. Add remaining ingredients; bring to a boil. Reduce heat and simmer, uncovered, for 2-3 hours. Discard bay leaves before serving. **Yield:** 14 servings (3-1/2 quarts).

Exchanges: 1-1/2 Vegetable, 1 Starch, 1 Lean Meat

Nutritional Information

Serving Size: 1 cup
Calories: 163
Sodium: 53 mg
Cholesterol: 20 mg

Carbohydrate: 28 gm
Protein: 14 gm
Fat: trace
Fiber: 6 gm

Hearty Split Pea Soup

Barbara Link, Alta Loma, California

*For a different spin on traditional split pea soup, try this recipe.
The flavor is peppery rather than smoky, and
the corned beef is an unexpected, tasty change of pace.*

1 bag (1 pound) dry split peas
8 cups water
**2 medium potatoes, peeled and
    cubed**
2 large onions, chopped
2 medium carrots, chopped
**2 cups cubed cooked corned beef
    or ham**
1/2 cup chopped celery
**5 teaspoons low-sodium chicken
    bouillon granules**
1 teaspoon dried marjoram
1 teaspoon poultry seasoning
1 teaspoon rubbed sage
1 teaspoon pepper
1/2 teaspoon dried basil
1/2 teaspoon salt-free seasoning blend

In a Dutch oven or soup kettle, combine
all ingredients; bring to a boil. Reduce
heat; cover and simmer for 1-1/4 to 1-1/2
hours or until peas and vegetables are tender. **Yield:** 12 servings (3 quarts).

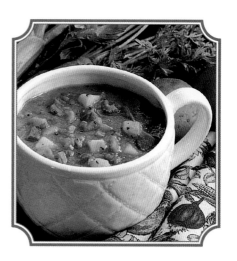

Exchanges: 2 Starch, 1 Lean Meat, 1 Vegetable, 1 Fat

Nutritional Information

Serving Size: 1 cup
Calories: 278
Sodium: 495 mg
Cholesterol: 39 mg

Carbohydrate: 34 gm
Protein: 19 gm
Fat: 8 gm
Fiber: 11 gm

Rainy Day Soup

Laine Fengarinas, Palm Harbor, Florida

One rainy day a few years back, this comforting soup was served at a local arts and crafts bazaar. Now family members request it when they're feeling blue.

1 pound ground turkey breast
1 can (46 ounces) low-sodium V-8 juice
1 jar (16 ounces) thick and chunky salsa
1 can (14-1/2 ounces) low-sodium chicken broth
1 can (16 ounces) kidney beans, rinsed and drained
1 package (10 ounces) frozen mixed vegetables
4 cups shredded cabbage
1 cup chopped onion
1/2 cup cubed peeled potatoes
1/3 cup medium pearl barley

In a Dutch oven or soup kettle coated with nonstick cooking spray, brown turkey over medium heat; drain. Add remaining ingredients; bring to a boil. Reduce heat; cover and simmer for 60-70 minutes or until the vegetables and barley are tender. **Yield:** 12 servings (3 quarts).

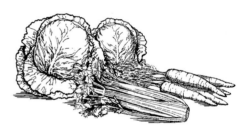

Exchanges: 2 Vegetable, 1 Starch, 1 Lean Meat

Nutritional Information

Serving Size: 1 cup
Calories: 184
Sodium: 408 mg
Cholesterol: 24 mg

Carbohydrate: 28 gm
Protein: 15 gm
Fat: 1 gm
Fiber: 7 gm

Harvest Turkey Soup

Linda Sand, Winsted, Connecticut

Herbs and spices make dishes like this taste terrific.
It also has a colorful blend of vegetables.

1 turkey carcass (from a
   12-pound turkey)
5 quarts water
2 large carrots, shredded
1 cup chopped celery
1 large onion, chopped
4 low-sodium chicken bouillon
   cubes
2 cans (14 ounces *each*) no-salt-
   added stewed tomatoes
3/4 cup fresh *or* frozen peas
3/4 cup long grain rice
1 package (10 ounces) frozen
   chopped spinach
1 tablespoon salt-free seasoning
   blend
3/4 teaspoon pepper
1/2 teaspoon dried marjoram
1/2 teaspoon dried thyme

Place the turkey carcass and water in a Dutch oven or soup kettle; bring to a boil. Reduce heat; cover and simmer for 1-1/2 hours. Remove carcass; allow to cool. Remove turkey from bones and cut into bite-size pieces; set aside. Strain broth. Add carrots, celery, onion and bouillon; bring to a boil. Reduce heat; cover and simmer for 30 minutes. Add the tomatoes, peas, rice, spinach, seasoning blend, pepper, marjoram, thyme and reserved turkey. Return to a boil; cook, uncovered, for 20 minutes or until rice is tender. **Yield:** 22 servings (5-1/2 quarts).

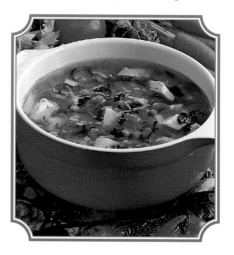

Exchanges: 1 Lean Meat, 1 Vegetable, 1/2 Starch

Nutritional Information

Serving Size: 1 cup
Calories: 94
Sodium: 65 mg
Cholesterol: 24 mg

Carbohydrate: 11 gm
Protein: 11 gm
Fat: 1 gm
Fiber: 2 gm
(Calculated with 22 ounces meat)

Garden Harvest Chili

Debbie Cosford, Bayfield, Ontario

Anytime you're looking for a way to use up your zucchini and squash, this recipe gives a different taste sensation. My husband really enjoys this chili.

1 medium sweet red pepper, chopped
1 medium onion, chopped
4 garlic cloves, minced
2 tablespoons vegetable oil
1 tablespoon chili powder
1 teaspoon ground cumin
1 teaspoon dried oregano
2 cups cubed peeled butternut squash
2 cans (14-1/2 ounces *each*) no-salt-added tomatoes, undrained and cut up
2 cups diced zucchini
1 can (15 ounces) black beans, rinsed and drained
1 cup frozen corn
1/4 cup minced fresh parsley

In a 3-qt. saucepan, saute red pepper, onion and garlic in oil until tender. Stir in chili powder, cumin, oregano, butternut squash and tomatoes; bring to a boil. Reduce heat; cover and simmer for 10-15 minutes or until squash is almost tender. Stir in remaining ingredients; cover and simmer 10 minutes more. **Yield:** 7 servings (1-3/4 quarts).

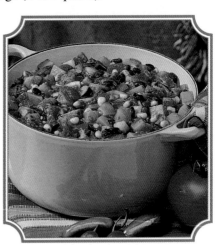

Exchanges: 2-1/2 Vegetable, 1 Starch, 1/2 Fat

Nutritional Information

Serving Size: 1 cup
Calories: 169
Sodium: 205 mg
Cholesterol: 0 mg

Carbohydrate: 28 gm
Protein: 7 gm
Fat: 5 gm
Fiber: 8 gm

Sausage Soup

Sonya Atkins, Farmington, Missouri

I created this soup by adapting one of my mother-in-law's recipes. It originally called for pork sausage, but I substitute turkey sausage with great results.

1 pound bulk turkey breakfast sausage
1 cup chopped onion
3 cups water
2 low-sodium chicken bouillon cubes
4 cups cubed peeled potatoes
1/2 teaspoon salt-free seasoning blend
1/4 teaspoon pepper
1/4 teaspoon dried sage
2 cups frozen corn
1 can (15 ounces) cream-style corn
1-1/2 cups evaporated skim milk
2/3 cup chopped sweet red pepper

In a soup kettle or Dutch oven over medium heat, cook sausage and onion until sausage is no longer pink and onion is tender; drain. Add water and bouillon; bring to a boil. Add potatoes, seasoning blend, pepper and sage; return to a boil. Reduce heat; cover and simmer for 25-30 minutes or until potatoes are tender. Stir in corn and evaporated milk; heat through. Garnish with red pepper. **Yield:** 10 servings (2-1/2 quarts).

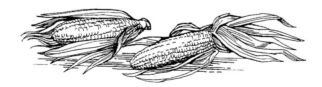

Exchanges: 1-1/2 Starch, 1-1/2 Lean Meat, 1/2 Vegetable, 1/2 Fat

Nutritional Information

Serving Size: 1 cup
Calories: 269
Sodium: 519 mg
Cholesterol: 39 mg

Carbohydrate: 34 gm
Protein: 17 gm
Fat: 8 gm
Fiber: 3 gm

Green Bean Soup

Elvira Beckenhauer, Omaha, Nebraska

This soup has been passed down for generations beginning with my great-grandmother. I make it often, especially when I can use homegrown beans, carrots, onions and potatoes.

1 quart water
2 cups fresh green beans, cut into 2-inch pieces
1-1/2 cups cubed peeled potatoes
1 cup cubed fully cooked low-sodium ham
1/2 cup thinly sliced carrot
1 medium onion, diced
1 bay leaf
1 sprig fresh parsley
1 sprig fresh savory *or* 1/4 teaspoon dried savory
1 low-sodium beef bouillon cube
1/4 teaspoon pepper
1/2 teaspoon salt-free seasoning blend

In a 2-qt. saucepan, combine all ingredients; bring to a boil. Reduce heat; cover and simmer for 20 minutes or until vegetables are tender. Before serving, discard bay leaf and parsley and savory sprigs. **Yield:** 6 servings.

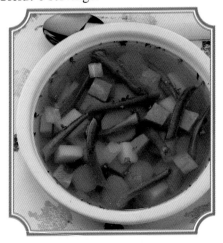

Exchanges: 1 Lean Meat, 1 Vegetable, 1/2 Starch

Nutritional Information

Serving Size: 1 cup
Calories: 121
Sodium: 387 mg
Cholesterol: 20 mg

Carbohydrate: 15 gm
Protein: 11 gm
Fat: 2 gm
Fiber: 2 gm

Herbed Fish Soup

Geraldine De Iure, Calgary, Alberta

My husband loves fish prepared in a variety of ways, so it's no surprise this soup has become one of his most-requested meals. I think you'll also enjoy its comforting flavor.

1 pound frozen fish fillets (cod, haddock, etc.), partially thawed
1 cup diced carrots
1 cup sliced fresh mushrooms
1 medium onion, sliced
1 garlic clove, minced
2 tablespoons vegetable oil
1/2 cup all-purpose flour
1/4 teaspoon dried thyme
1/4 teaspoon dill weed
Dash pepper
4 cups low-sodium chicken broth
1 bay leaf
1-1/2 cups frozen cut green beans

Cut fish into bite-size pieces; set aside. In a saucepan, saute carrots, mushrooms, onion and garlic in oil until onion is tender. Stir in flour, thyme, dill and pepper until smooth. Stir in broth; bring to a boil. Add bay leaf. Reduce heat; cover and simmer for 12-15 minutes or until carrots are tender. Add fish and beans. Simmer, uncovered, for 5 minutes or until fish is opaque and flakes easily. Discard bay leaf. **Yield:** 7 servings (about 2 quarts).

Exchanges: 1-1/2 Lean Meat, 1 Vegetable, 1 Fat, 1/2 Starch

Nutritional Information

Serving Size: 1/7 recipe
Calories: 166
Sodium: 105 mg
Cholesterol: 30 mg

Carbohydrate: 14 gm
Protein: 15 gm
Fat: 5 gm
Fiber: 2 gm

Carrot Apple Soup

Ruby Williams, Bogalusa, Louisiana

*On a brisk fall day, nothing is more appealing than a
steaming bowl of this soup. Even though
it's lower in fat, it still has old-time goodness.*

1 tablespoon reduced-fat
  margarine
8 medium carrots, thinly sliced
2 medium tart apples, peeled and
  chopped
1 medium onion, chopped
1 celery rib, thinly sliced
5 cups low-sodium chicken broth
1/2 teaspoon rubbed sage
1/4 teaspoon pepper
1 bay leaf

In a large saucepan, melt the margarine. Add carrots, apples, onion and celery; cook and stir until onion is tender, about 5 minutes. Add broth, sage, pepper and bay leaf; bring to a boil. Reduce heat; cover and simmer for 20 minutes or until carrots are tender. Discard bay leaf. Cool soup for 5 minutes. Puree one-third at a time in a blender or food processor. Return to the saucepan; cover and cook over medium until heated through. **Yield:** 7 servings.

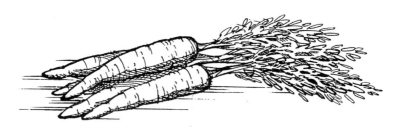

Exchanges: 2 Vegetable, 1/2 Starch

Nutritional Information

Serving Size: 1 cup
Calories: 97
Sodium: 147 mg
Cholesterol: 3 mg

Carbohydrate: 17 gm
Protein: 4 gm
Fat: 2 gm
Fiber: 4 gm

Cream of Tomato Soup

Gail Harris, Ramer, Tennessee

This fresh-tasting soup is the first recipe I learned in my high-school home economics class. I've fixed it quite often since then. It's wonderful made with ripe garden tomatoes.

2-1/2 cups diced peeled tomatoes
1/4 cup diced celery
1/4 cup diced onion
1 tablespoon vegetable oil
2 tablespoons all-purpose flour
1 cup evaporated skim milk
1 teaspoon salt-free seasoning blend
1/8 teaspoon pepper
3 tablespoons nonfat sour cream
3 teaspoons minced fresh parsley

In a saucepan, combine tomatoes, celery and onion; bring to a boil. Reduce heat; cover and simmer for 15 minutes, stirring often. Cool for 10 minutes; pour into a blender. Cover and process until smooth. In a large saucepan, heat oil; stir in flour until smooth. Gradually add milk; bring to a boil. Cook and stir for 2 minutes. Gradually stir in tomato mixture. Add seasoning blend and pepper; heat through. Top individual servings with sour cream and parsley. **Yield:** 3 servings (3-1/2 cups).

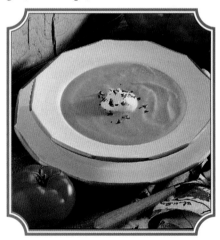

Exchanges: 2 Vegetable, 1 Skim Milk, 1 Fat

Nutritional Information

Serving Size: 1/3 recipe
Calories: 184
Sodium: 134 mg
Cholesterol: 4 mg

Carbohydrate: 26 gm
Protein: 10 gm
Fat: 5 gm
Fiber: 2 gm

Summer Garden Soup

Patsy Bell Hobson, Liberty, Missouri

*This soup is very tasty, and the best part is
that all of the main ingredients come straight from
your garden. It's even good when served chilled.*

1 cup chopped onion
4 to 6 garlic cloves, minced
2 tablespoons olive *or*
  vegetable oil
3 cups chopped fresh tomatoes
1 cup fresh *or* frozen cut green
  beans
1 tablespoon minced fresh basil
  or 1 teaspoon dried basil
1 teaspoon minced fresh
  tarragon *or* 1/4 teaspoon dried
  tarragon
1/2 teaspoon minced fresh dill
  or pinch dill weed
1/4 teaspoon pepper
1/4 teaspoon salt-free seasoning
  blend
3-1/2 cups low-sodium chicken broth
1 cup fresh *or* frozen peas
1 cup sliced zucchini *or* yellow
  summer squash

In a saucepan, saute onion and garlic in oil
until onion is tender. Add the tomatoes,
beans, basil, tarragon, dill, pepper and
seasoning blend; simmer for 10 minutes.
Add broth, peas and zucchini; simmer
for 5-10 minutes or until vegetables are
crisp-tender. **Yield:** 8 servings (2 quarts).

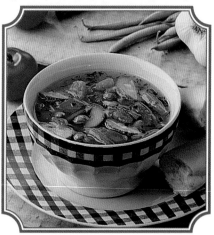

Exchanges: 1-1/2 Vegetable, 1 Fat
Nutritional Information

Serving Size: 1 cup
Calories: 92
Sodium: 76 mg
Cholesterol: 2 mg

Carbohydrate: 11 gm
Protein: 4 gm
Fat: 5 gm
Fiber: 3 gm

Vegetable Bean Chili

Rene Fry, Hampstead, Maryland

*Because it is so hearty, no one misses the meat in this chili.
Both family and friends ask me to make it often*

1 medium zucchini, sliced 1/4
inch thick
1 medium green pepper,
chopped
1 cup chopped onion
1 cup shredded carrots
1/2 cup finely chopped celery
2 garlic cloves, minced
1/4 cup olive *or* vegetable oil
2 cans (14-1/2 ounces *each*) no-salt-
added tomatoes, undrained, cut up
1 jar (8 ounces) picante sauce
1 teaspoon low-sodium beef
bouillon granules
1-1/2 teaspoons ground cumin
1 can (15-1/2 ounces) chili
beans, undrained
1 can (15 ounces) garbanzo
beans, rinsed and drained
1 can (2-1/4 ounces) sliced ripe
olives, drained

In a 4-qt. kettle or Dutch oven, saute zucchini, green pepper, onion, carrots, celery and garlic in oil until tender. Stir in tomatoes, picante sauce, bouillon and cumin; bring to a boil. Reduce heat; simmer, uncovered, for 30 minutes, stirring occasionally. Add beans and olives; heat through. **Yield:** 9 servings (2-1/4 quarts).

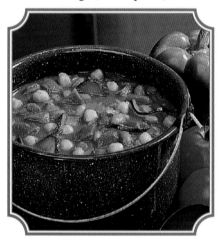

Exchanges: 2 Vegetable, 1-1/2 Starch, 1-1/2 Fat, 1/2 Lean Meat

Nutritional Information

Serving Size: 1 cup
Calories: 211
Sodium: 647 mg
Cholesterol: trace

Carbohydrate: 30 gm
Protein: 7 gm
Fat: 8 gm
Fiber: 7 gm

Tortellini Soup

Karen Rago, Bristol, Pennsylvania

This soup is filling and easy to prepare. It makes a fresh-tasting and satisfying first course or light meal in itself.

1 medium onion, chopped
1 garlic clove, minced
2 cans (14-1/2 ounces *each***) low-sodium chicken broth**
8 ounces refrigerated cheese tortellini
1 can (14-1/2 ounces) no-salt-added stewed tomatoes
1 package (10 ounces) frozen chopped spinach, thawed and drained

In a large saucepan coated with nonstick cooking spray, saute onion and garlic until tender. Add broth; bring to a boil. Add the tortellini; reduce heat. Simmer for 10 minutes or until tortellini is tender. Stir in tomatoes and spinach; heat through. **Yield:** 7 servings.

DRAINING FROZEN SPINACH. To remove excess moisture from thawed frozen spinach, hold it over the sink and squeeze it with your hands. Then sandwich the spinach between layers of paper towel and press out any remaining liquid.

Exchanges: 1-1/2 Vegetable, 1 Starch, 1/2 Lean Meat

Nutritional Information

Serving Size: 1/7 recipe
Calories: 159
Sodium: 197 mg
Cholesterol: 14 mg

Carbohydrate: 23 gm
Protein: 9 gm
Fat: 3 gm
Fiber: 3 gm

Beef

If you want to offer your family and friends a down-home dinner, nothing can compare to a meaty main course featuring ground beef or a tender beef cut.

Italian Beef Sandwiches

Margery Bryan, Royal City, Washington

Everyone enjoys these hearty, tasty sandwiches that can be made for two—or any size group.

3 garlic cloves, *divided*
2 cups low-sodium beef broth
1/2 teaspoon dried oregano, *divided*
1 small onion, sliced
1 small green pepper, cut into strips
1 tablespoon vegetable oil
2 beef tip *or* sandwich steaks (1/4 inch thick)
2 Italian rolls, split

Cut one garlic clove in half; place in a saucepan. Add broth and 1/4 teaspoon oregano; cook over medium-low heat for 10 minutes. Discard garlic clove. Remove broth from the heat and set aside. Mince remaining garlic; place in a skillet. Add the onion, green pepper, oil and remaining oregano; cook and stir over medium heat until crisp-tender. Remove vegetables and keep warm. Add meat to the skillet; cook over medium heat until browned on both sides. Add reserved broth; simmer for 10-12 minutes or until meat is tender. To serve, brush cut sides of rolls with some of the broth; top with meat and vegetables. **Yield:** 2 servings.

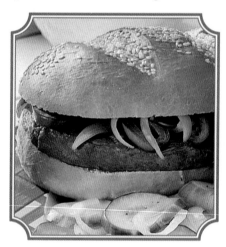

Exchanges: 3-1/2 Lean Meat, 2-1/2 Starch, 2 Vegetable, 1 Fat

Nutritional Information

Serving Size: 1 sandwich
Calories: 500
Sodium: 493 mg
Cholesterol: 68 mg

Carbohydrate: 49 gm
Protein: 38 gm
Fat: 17 gm
Fiber: 4 gm

Mexi-Corn Lasagna

Darlene Clayton, Danbury, Wisconsin

Tortillas and a spicy meat sauce plus the corn make this lasagna out of the ordinary! I like to serve it with a salad and corn bread.

1 pound lean ground beef
2 cups fresh *or* frozen corn
2 cans (8 ounces *each*) no-salt-added tomato sauce
1 cup picante sauce
1 tablespoon chili powder
1-1/2 teaspoons ground cumin
10 flour tortillas (7 inches)
2 cups low-fat cottage cheese
Egg substitute equivalent to 2 eggs
2 tablespoons grated Parmesan cheese
1 teaspoon dried oregano
1/2 teaspoon garlic powder
1 cup (4 ounces) reduced-fat shredded cheddar cheese

In a skillet, cook beef over medium heat until no longer pink; drain. Add corn, tomato sauce, picante sauce, chili powder and cumin; bring to a boil. Reduce heat; cover and simmer for 5 minutes. Place half of the tortillas in the bottom and up the sides of a 13-in. x 9-in. x 2-in. baking pan coated with nonstick cooking spray. Spoon meat mixture over tortillas. Combine cottage cheese, egg substitute, Parmesan, oregano and garlic powder; spread over meat mixture. Top with remaining tortillas. Cover and bake at 375° for 30 minutes. Sprinkle with cheese; return to the oven for 10 minutes or until cheese is melted. **Yield:** 12 servings.

Exchanges: 2-1/2 Lean Meat, 1-1/2 Starch, 1/2 Fat

Nutritional Information

Serving Size: 1/12 recipe
Calories: 294
Sodium: 635 mg
Cholesterol: 20 mg

Carbohydrate: 33 gm
Protein: 22 gm
Fat: 8 gm
Fiber: 1 gm

Old-Fashioned Beef Stew

Anne Heinonen, Howell, Michigan

This rich, hearty beef stew has a garden full of flavor with vegetables like cabbage, rutabaga and carrots. You can also throw in extra vegetables to stretch it.

1 boneless chuck roast (2 pounds), cut into 1/2-inch cubes
1 tablespoon vegetable oil
1 large onion, chopped
4 cups water
1 teaspoon salt-free seasoning blend
1/2 teaspoon pepper
5 to 6 medium potatoes, peeled and cut into 1/2-inch cubes
5 medium carrots, cut into 1/4-inch slices
1 medium rutabaga, peeled and cut into 1/2-inch cubes
1 cup sliced celery (1/2-inch pieces)
1/2 medium head cabbage, finely sliced
1/3 cup all-purpose flour
1 cup cold water
2 teaspoons browning sauce

In a Dutch oven over medium-high heat, brown meat in oil. Add onion, water, seasoning blend and pepper; bring to a boil. Reduce heat; cover and simmer for 2 hours. Add the vegetables; cover and simmer for 30 minutes or until the meat and vegetables are tender. Combine flour, cold water and browning sauce until smooth. Stir into stew; bring to a boil, stirring constantly. Boil for 2 minutes or until thickened. **Yield:** 8 servings.

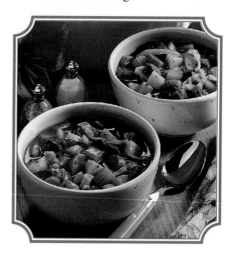

Exchanges: 3-1/2 Lean Meat, 2 Vegetable, 1 Starch
Nutritional Information
Serving Size: 1-1/2 cups
Calories: 359
Sodium: 218 mg
Cholesterol: 82 mg

Carbohydrate: 35 gm
Protein: 30 gm
Fat: 12 gm
Fiber: 6 gm

Pepper Steak

Jean Bunders, Wauzeka, Wisconsin

I attended a cooking class a few years ago, and this was one of the recipes we learned to prepare. When I tried it at home, my family raved about the delicious flavor.

1 pound boneless sirloin steak
1 tablespoon vegetable oil
1 garlic clove, minced
1 teaspoon ground ginger
1 teaspoon salt-free seasoning blend
1/2 teaspoon pepper
3 large green peppers, thinly sliced
2 large onions, thinly sliced
3/4 teaspoon low-sodium beef bouillon granules
3/4 cup hot water
1 can (8 ounces) sliced water chestnuts, drained
1 tablespoon cornstarch
1/4 cup light soy sauce
1/4 cup cold water
1/2 teaspoon sugar

Cut steak into 2-in. x 1/8-in. strips. In a large nonstick skillet or wok, brown steak in oil. Add garlic, ginger, seasoning blend and pepper; cook 1 minute. Remove meat and keep warm. Add green peppers and onions to skillet; cook and stir for 5 minutes or until crisp-tender. Dissolve bouillon in hot water; add to skillet with water chestnuts. Combine cornstarch, soy sauce, cold water and sugar until smooth; stir into skillet. Add meat. Cook and stir until mixture boils; cook and stir 2 minutes more. **Yield:** 6 servings.

SLICING PEPPERS. Wash peppers thoroughly, then cut in half vertically from one stem end to the other. Pull out the seed core and wash the inside of the pepper. For easier slicing, cut from the flesh side instead of from the tougher skin side.

Exchanges: 2-1/2 Lean Meat, 2 Vegetable
Nutritional Information
Serving Size: 1/6 recipe
Calories: 185
Sodium: 666 mg
Cholesterol: 45 mg

Carbohydrate: 12 gm
Protein: 18 gm
Fat: 7 gm
Fiber: 3 gm

Steak 'n' Gravy

Betty Janway, Ruston, Louisiana

Slow cooking in a zesty tomato sauce for hours helps the round steak become nice and tender. This nicely spiced steak with gravy makes a satisfying meal served over rice or mashed potatoes.

1 pound round steak, trimmed
1 tablespoon vegetable oil
1-1/2 cups water
1 can (8 ounces) no-salt-added
   tomato sauce
1 teaspoon ground cumin
1 teaspoon garlic powder
1/2 teaspoon salt-free seasoning blend
1/4 teaspoon pepper
2 tablespoons all-purpose flour
1/4 cup cold water
2 cups mashed potatoes

Cut beef into bite-size pieces. In a non-stick skillet, brown meat in oil. Transfer to a slow cooker. Cover with water; add tomato sauce and seasonings. Cover and cook on low for 8 hours, or on high for 4 hours, or until meat is tender. In a small bowl, combine flour and cold water until smooth; stir into liquid in slow cooker. Cover and cook on high 30 minutes longer or until gravy is thickened. Serve over potatoes. **Yield:** 4 servings.

> **MAKING MASHED POTATOES.** Cook the potatoes only until they're fork-tender. Drain immediately so they don't absorb excess moisture. Beat the potatoes until they're light and fluffy. Overbeating will turn them sticky and starchy.

Exchanges: 3-1/2 Lean Meat, 1-1/2 Starch, 1 Fat

Nutritional Information

Serving Size: 1/4 recipe
Calories: 361
Sodium: 336 mg
Cholesterol: 72 mg

Carbohydrate: 26 gm
Protein: 28 gm
Fat: 16 gm
Fiber: 1 gm

Enchilada Casserole

Nancy VanderVeer, Knoxville, Iowa

I get great reviews every time I serve this—
even from my father, who usually doesn't like Mexican food.

1 pound lean ground beef
1 can (10 ounces) enchilada sauce
1 cup salsa
6 flour tortillas (10 inch)
2 cups frozen corn
3 cups (12 ounces) shredded
  reduced-fat cheddar cheese

In a skillet, cook beef over medium heat until no longer pink; drain. Stir in enchilada sauce and salsa; set aside. Place two tortillas, overlapping as necessary, in the bottom of a 13-in. x 9-in. x 2-in. baking dish coated with nonstick cooking spray. Cover with one-third of the meat mixture; top with 1 cup corn; sprinkle with 1 cup cheese. Repeat layers once, then top with remaining tortillas, meat and cheese.

Bake, uncovered, at 350° for 30 minutes or until bubbly. **Yield:** 8 servings.

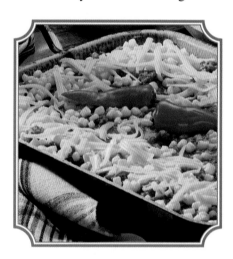

Exchanges: 3 Meat, 1-1/2 Starch, 1 Fat

Nutritional Information

Serving Size: 1/8 recipe
Calories: 323
Sodium: 878 mg
Cholesterol: 30 mg

Carbohydrate: 29 gm
Protein: 26 gm
Fat: 12 gm
Fiber: 2 gm

Green Chili Stew

Mary Spill, Tierra Amarilla, New Mexico

*Peppers give this down–home stew a
wonderful rich flavor your family will love.*

1 pound lean ground beef
1 pound ground pork
8 to 10 Anaheim chilies,
   roasted, peeled and chopped
   or 3 cans (4 ounces *each*)
   chopped green chilies
4 medium potatoes, peeled and
   diced
2 cans (14-1/2 ounces *each*) no-
   salt-added tomatoes, undrained
   and cut up
2 cups water
1 garlic clove, minced
1 teaspoon salt-free seasoning
   blend
1/2 teaspoon dried oregano
1/4 teaspoon pepper
1/4 teaspoon dried coriander

In a large kettle or Dutch oven, brown beef
and pork until no longer pink; drain. Add
remaining ingredients. Cover and simmer
for 45 minutes. **Yield:** 10 servings.

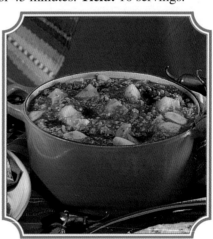

Exchanges: 2-1/2 Meat, 1 Vegetable, 1/2 Starch

Nutritional Information

Serving Size: 1/8 recipe
Calories: 258
Sodium: 191 mg
Cholesterol: 49 mg

Carbohydrate: 15 gm
Protein: 19 gm
Fat: 14 gm
Fiber: 3 gm

Hobo Dinner

Pat Walter, Pine Island, Minnesota

In this recipe, the meat and vegetables all cook together wrapped in a piece of foil. This single-serving supper is a favorite. I especially like the fact that there is little cleanup.

1/4 pound lean ground beef
1 potato, sliced
1 carrot, sliced
2 tablespoons chopped onion
1/8 teaspoon salt-free seasoning blend
Pepper to taste

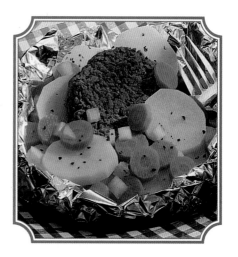

Shape beef into a patty; place in the center of a large piece of heavy-duty foil (18 in. x 13 in.). Add potato, carrot and onion. Sprinkle with seasoning blend and pepper. Fold foil over and seal well; place on a baking sheet. Bake at 350° for 45 minutes. Open foil carefully. **Yield:** 1 serving. **Editor's Note:** Dinner may also be grilled, covered, over medium heat for 45-60 minutes or until potato is tender.

Exchanges: 3 Lean Meat, 2 Vegetable, 1-1/2 Starch

Nutritional Information

Serving Size: 1 recipe
Calories: 368
Sodium: 168 mg
Cholesterol: 41 mg

Carbohydrate: 44 gm
Protein: 27 gm
Fat: 10 gm
Fiber: 6 gm

Yankee Pot Roast

Bill Schiltz, Walden, New York

*Rubbing garlic onto the roast before browning adds lots of flavor.
With this recipe, the meat and vegetables turn out moist and tender.*

2 garlic cloves, minced
1 beef eye of round roast
(3 pounds)
1/4 cup all-purpose flour
2 tablespoons vegetable oil
1 cup low-sodium tomato juice
4 medium carrots, sliced
2 medium onions, chopped
1 cup thinly sliced celery
2 bay leaves
1 teaspoon salt-free seasoning
blend
1/2 teaspoon dried thyme
1/4 teaspoon pepper
4 medium potatoes, peeled and
quartered

Rub garlic onto roast, then coat with flour. In a large Dutch oven, brown roast in oil. Add tomato juice, carrots, onions, celery, bay leaves, seasoning blend, thyme and pepper; bring to a boil. Reduce heat; cover and simmer for 3-1/2 hours, turning meat occasionally. Add potatoes; simmer for 30 minutes or until tender. Discard bay leaves. Remove roast and slice; serve with vegetables and gravy. **Yield:** 12 servings.

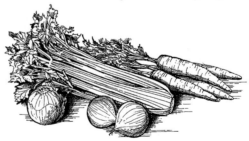

Exchanges: 3-1/2 Lean Meat, 1-1/2 Fat, 1 Vegetable, 1/2 Starch

Nutritional Information

Serving Size: 1/12 recipe
Calories: 260
Sodium: 92 mg
Cholesterol: 66 mg

Carbohydrate: 14 gm
Protein: 29 gm
Fat: 10 gm
Fiber: 2 gm

Savory Braised Beef

Eva Knight, Nashua, New Hampshire

Everyone will enjoy this delicious dish. With meat, potatoes and vegetables, it's a meal in itself.

1/2 pound boneless chuck roast
3/4 cup water
  1 small apple, thinly sliced
  1 small onion, thinly sliced
1/4 teaspoon salt-free seasoning blend
1/4 teaspoon pepper
  4 small new potatoes, halved
  2 cabbage wedges (about 2 inches thick)
  1 can (14-1/2 ounces) no-salt-added stewed tomatoes
1-1/2 teaspoons cornstarch
1-1/2 teaspoons water

Trim fat from meat and cut into 1-in. cubes; brown in a skillet coated with non-stick cooking spray. Add water, apple, onion, seasoning blend and pepper. Cover and simmer for 1-1/4 hours. Add potatoes and cabbage; cover and simmer for 35 minutes or until vegetables are tender. Stir in tomatoes; cover and simmer for 10 minutes. Combine cornstarch and water until smooth; stir into skillet. Bring to a boil; cook and stir for 2 minutes. **Yield:** 2 servings.

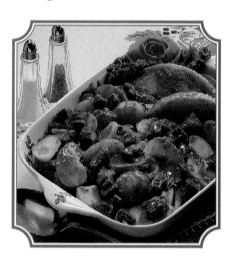

Exchanges: 3 Lean Meat, 2 Vegetable, 2 Starch, 1 Fruit

Nutritional Information

Serving Size: 1/2 recipe
Calories: 469
Sodium: 94 mg
Cholesterol: 75 mg

Carbohydrate: 68 gm
Protein: 30 gm
Fat: 11 gm
Fiber: 13 gm

Beef Rouladen

Karin Cousineau, Burlington, North Carolina

When Mother made meat for a Sunday dinner, it was a terrific treat. My favorite is this tender beef dish, which gets its great flavor from Dijon mustard.

1/4 cup Dijon mustard
   8 slices top round steak, 1/4 inch thick (2 pounds)
1/4 teaspoon salt-free seasoning blend
Pepper to taste
   8 turkey bacon strips
   1 large onion, cut into thin wedges
   1 tablespoon vegetable oil
   3 cups low-sodium beef broth
1/3 cup all-purpose flour
1/2 cup water
   1 tablespoon chopped fresh parsley

Lightly spread mustard on each slice of steak; sprinkle with seasoning blend and pepper. Place 1 bacon strip and a few onion wedges on each slice; roll up and secure with toothpicks. Brown in a nonstick skillet in oil; drain. Add broth; bring to a boil. Reduce heat; cover and simmer for 1-1/2 hours or until meat is tender. Remove meat and keep warm. Combine flour and water until smooth; stir into broth. Bring to a boil. Cook and stir for 2 minutes or until thickened. Remove toothpicks from meat and return to gravy; heat through. Sprinkle with parsley. **Yield:** 8 servings.

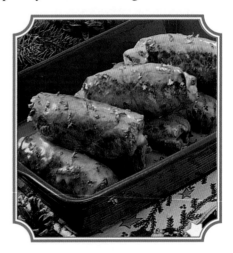

Exchanges: 4 Lean Meat, 1 Fat, 1/2 Starch

Nutritional Information

Serving Size: 1 piece
Calories: 299
Sodium: 458 mg
Cholesterol: 82 mg

Carbohydrate: 7 gm
Protein: 30 gm
Fat: 16 gm
Fiber: trace

Shamrock Stew

Robin Perry, Seneca, Pennsylvania

You don't have to be Irish to enjoy this savory stew.
Homemade dumplings make it extra special.

1/4 cup all-purpose flour
3/4 teaspoon salt-free seasoning blend
1/4 teaspoon pepper
2 pounds round steak, cut into 1-inch cubes
1 tablespoon vegetable oil
1 can (8 ounces) no-salt-added tomato sauce
2 cups water
1 large onion, sliced
1 teaspoon dried marjoram
1 bay leaf
1 pound carrots, cut into 1-inch pieces
1 package (10 ounces) frozen peas
DUMPLINGS:
1 cup all-purpose flour
1 teaspoon baking powder
1/4 cup skim milk
1 egg, beaten
1 tablespoon vegetable oil
1 tablespoon chopped fresh parsley

In a medium bowl, combine flour, seasoning blend and pepper; set aside 2 tablespoons. Add meat to bowl and toss to coat. In a 6-qt. Dutch oven over medium heat, brown the meat in oil. Stir in tomato sauce, water and reserved flour mixture. Add onion, marjoram and bay leaf; bring to a boil. Reduce heat; cover and simmer for 2 hours, stirring occasionally. Add carrots; cover and simmer for 45 minutes. Stir in peas. Cover and simmer for 15 minutes or until the vegetables are tender. Discard bay leaf. For dumplings, combine flour and baking powder. Stir in milk, egg, oil and parsley. Drop by tablespoonfuls onto simmering stew. Cover and cook for 12-14 minutes or until done (do not lift the cover while simmering). Serve immediately. **Yield:** 8 servings.

Exchanges: 3-1/2 Lean Meat, 2 Vegetable, 1 Starch, 1 Fat

Nutritional Information

Serving Size: 1/8 recipe
Calories: 386
Sodium: 162 mg
Cholesterol: 96 mg

Carbohydrate: 31 gm
Protein: 31 gm
Fat: 15 gm
Fiber: 5 gm

Fabulous Fajitas

Janie Reitz, Rochester, Minnesota

When friends call to ask me for a new recipe to try, I often suggest these flavorful fajitas. Just put the beef in the slow cooker before church and come home to a hot delicious main dish.

1-1/2 pounds boneless sirloin
    steak, cut into thin strips
1 tablespoon vegetable oil
2 tablespoons lemon juice
1 garlic clove, minced
1-1/2 teaspoons ground cumin
1 teaspoon salt-free seasoning
    blend
1/2 teaspoon chili powder
1/4 to 1/2 teaspoon crushed red
    pepper flakes
1 large green pepper, julienned
1 large onion, julienned
8 flour tortillas (7 inches)
Shredded fat-free cheddar cheese,
    salsa, nonfat sour cream, lettuce
    and tomatoes, optional

In a nonstick skillet over medium heat, brown the steak in oil. Place steak and drippings in a slow cooker. Add lemon juice, garlic, cumin, seasoning blend, chili powder and red pepper flakes; mix well. Cover and cook on high for 2-1/2 to 3 hours or until meat is tender. Add green pepper and onion; cover and cook for 1 hour or until vegetables are tender. Warm tortillas according to package directions; spoon beef and vegetables down the center of tortillas. Top each with cheese, salsa, sour cream, lettuce and tomatoes if desired. Fold in sides of tortillas and serve immediately. **Yield:** 8 servings.

Exchanges: 2-1/2 Lean Meat, 1-1/2 Starch, 1/2 Vegetable

Nutritional Information

Serving Size: 1/8 recipe
Calories: 313
Sodium: 286 mg
Cholesterol: 50 mg

Carbohydrate: 31 gm
Protein: 23 gm
Fat: 10 gm
Fiber: 2 gm
(Calculated without toppings)

Party Beef Casserole

Kelly Hardgrave, Hartman, Arkansas

Economical and delicious round steak is used in this comforting casserole.

3 tablespoons all-purpose flour
1 teaspoon salt-free seasoning
   blend
1/2 teaspoon pepper
2 pounds boneless round steak,
   cut into 1/2-inch cubes
1 tablespoon vegetable oil
1 cup water
1/2 cup low-sodium beef broth
1 garlic clove, minced
1 tablespoon dried minced onion
1/2 teaspoon dried thyme
1/4 teaspoon dried rosemary,
   crushed
2 cups sliced fresh mushrooms
2 cups frozen peas, thawed
3 cups mashed potatoes (prepared
   with milk and margarine)
Paprika

In a large resealable plastic bag, combine flour, seasoning blend and pepper; add beef cubes and shake to coat. In a nonstick skillet over medium heat, brown beef in oil. Place beef and drippings in a shallow 2-1/2-qt. baking dish coated with nonstick cooking spray. To skillet, add water, broth, garlic, onion, thyme and rosemary; bring to a boil. Simmer, uncovered, for 5 minutes; stir in mushrooms. Pour over meat; mix well. Cover and bake at 350° for 1-1/2 to 1-3/4 hours or until beef is tender. Sprinkle peas over meat. Spread potatoes evenly over top. Sprinkle with paprika. Bake 15-20 minutes more. **Yield:** 8 servings.

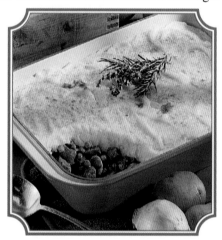

Exchanges: 3-1/2 Lean Meat, 1-1/2 Starch

Nutritional Information

Serving Size: 1/8 recipe
Calories: 339
Sodium: 307 mg
Cholesterol: 71 mg

Carbohydrate: 24 gm
Protein: 30 gm
Fat: 14 gm
Fiber: 2 gm

Mexican-Style Spaghetti

Mary Detweiler, West Farmington, Ohio

*A good friend shared this recipe with me. When my
family gets tired of the same old spaghetti, I like to serve this.
Cumin gives it an unusual taste twist.*

2 pounds lean ground beef
2 medium onions, chopped
1 medium green pepper, chopped
3 garlic cloves, minced
1 can (29 ounces) tomato puree
1 can (16 ounces) kidney beans,
**   rinsed and drained**
1 cup water
1/4 cup chopped fresh parsley
2 tablespoons chili powder
1 teaspoon ground cumin
1 teaspoon dried marjoram
1 teaspoon dried oregano
1 teaspoon salt-free seasoning
**   blend**
1/4 to 1/2 teaspoon cayenne pepper
1 package (12 ounces) spaghetti,
**   cooked and drained**

In a Dutch oven, brown beef, onions,
green pepper and garlic; drain. Add the
next 10 ingredients and mix well. Cover
and simmer for 2 hours, stirring occasionally. Serve over spaghetti. **Yield:** 8
servings.

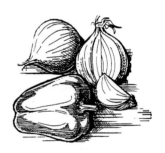

Exchanges: 3 Lean Meat, 3 Vegetable, 1-1/2 Starch

Nutritional Information

Serving Size: 1/8 recipe
Calories: 379
Sodium: 495 mg
Cholesterol: 41 mg

Carbohydrate: 39 gm
Protein: 32 gm
Fat: 11 gm
Fiber: 9 gm

Beef Cabbage Stew

Lesa Swartwood, Fulton, Missouri

This is one of my favorite meals since I don't have to stand over the stove or dirty a lot of pots and pans to prepare it. I often rely on this one-pot meal to feed my family of six.

1-1/2 pounds lean beef stew meat, cut into 1-inch pieces
2 low-sodium beef bouillon cubes
1 cup hot water
1 large onion, chopped
1/4 teaspoon pepper
1 bay leaf
2 medium potatoes, peeled and cubed
2 celery ribs, sliced
4 cups shredded cabbage
1 medium carrot, sliced
1 can (8 ounces) no-salt-added tomato sauce
1/4 teaspoon salt-free seasoning blend

In a large saucepan or Dutch oven, brown stew meat; drain. Meanwhile, dissolve bouillon cubes in water; add to beef. Add onion, pepper and bay leaf. Cover; simmer 1-1/4 hours or until meat is tender. Add potatoes, celery, cabbage and carrot. Cover and simmer 30 minutes or until vegetables are tender. Stir in tomato sauce and seasoning blend. Simmer, uncovered, 15-20 minutes more. Discard bay leaf before serving. **Yield:** 8 servings.

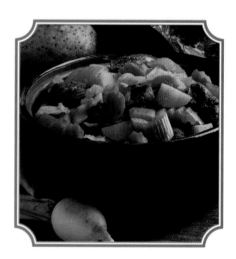

Exchanges: 3-1/2 Lean Meat, 1-1/2 Vegetable

Nutritional Information

Serving Size: 1/8 recipe
Calories: 272
Sodium: 313 mg
Cholesterol: 86 mg

Carbohydrate: 15 gm
Protein: 30 gm
Fat: 10 gm
Fiber: 3 gm

Broccoli Beef Curry

Andrea Su, Binghamton, New York

We developed our own version of this dish after tasting it at a local Indian restaurant. The curry is not overpowering—it has a wonderful flavor.

1-1/2 pounds round steak, cut into 1-inch cubes
2 to 3 garlic cloves, minced
2 teaspoons minced fresh gingerroot
1 teaspoon curry powder
1 teaspoon chili powder
1 teaspoon salt-free seasoning blend
2 large onions, diced
1 tablespoon vegetable oil
1 cup plus 2 tablespoons water, *divided*
1 pound fresh broccoli, cut into florets
2 teaspoons cornstarch
3 cups hot cooked rice

Toss meat with garlic, gingerroot, curry powder, chili powder and seasoning blend. In a large nonstick skillet or wok, cook meat and onions in oil until meat is browned. Stir in 1 cup water. Cover and simmer 1-1/2 hours or until beef is tender. Add broccoli; cover and cook until crisp-tender. Combine cornstarch and remaining water until smooth; add to skillet. Cook and stir for 2 minutes. Serve over rice. **Yield:** 6 servings.

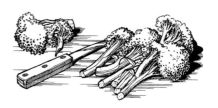

Exchanges: 3-1/2 Lean Meat, 2 Vegetable, 1 Starch

Nutritional Information

Serving Size: 1/6 recipe
Calories: 379
Sodium: 80 mg
Cholesterol: 69 mg

Carbohydrate: 35 gm
Protein: 30 gm
Fat: 14 gm
Fiber: 2 gm

Peppered Beef Tenderloin

Margaret Ninneman, La Crosse, Wisconsin
(ALSO PICTURED ON FRONT COVER)

When you're cooking for a crowd that really savors meat, this peppery, tempting tenderloin is perfect! It's important to let it rest for a few minutes before carving to allow the juices to work through the meat.

1 teaspoon dried oregano
1 teaspoon paprika
1 teaspoon dried thyme
1 teaspoon salt-free seasoning
  blend
1/2 teaspoon garlic powder
1/2 teaspoon onion powder
1/2 teaspoon pepper
1/2 teaspoon white pepper
1/8 to 1/4 teaspoon cayenne
  pepper
1 beef tenderloin (3 pounds)

Combine seasonings and rub over entire tenderloin. Place on a rack in a roasting pan. Bake, uncovered, at 425° until meat is cooked as desired. Allow approximately 45-50 minutes for rare or until a meat thermometer reads 140°, 55-60 minutes for medium-rare (150°), 62-65 minutes for medium (160°) and 67-70 minutes for well-done (170°). Let stand 10 min-

utes before carving. **Yield:** 12 servings.
Editor's Note: After seasoning, the uncooked tenderloin may be wrapped tightly and refrigerated overnight for a more intense flavor.

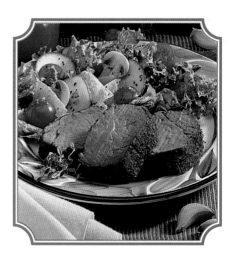

Exchanges: 4-1/2 Lean Meat

Nutritional Information

Serving Size: 1/12 recipe
Calories: 239
Sodium: 71 mg
Cholesterol: 95 mg

Carbohydrate: 0 gm
Protein: 32 gm
Fat: 11 gm
Fiber: 0 gm

Swiss Steak

Dianne Esposite, New Middleton, Ohio

*Mom was always glad to prepare this tender,
flavorful dish for a birthday dinner when I was growing up.
Now my family enjoys this entree.*

1/4 cup all-purpose flour
1 teaspoon salt-free seasoning
blend
1/4 teaspoon pepper
1-1/2 pounds round steak, trimmed
1 tablespoon vegetable oil
1 cup chopped celery
1 cup chopped onion
1/2 pound fresh mushrooms, sliced
1 cup water
1 garlic clove, minced
1 tablespoon steak sauce

Combine flour, seasoning blend and pepper. Cut steak into serving-size pieces; dredge in flour mixture. In a nonstick skillet, brown steak in oil. Drain and place in a 2-1/2-qt. casserole. Top with celery, onion and mushrooms. Combine water, garlic and steak sauce; pour over vegetables. Cover and bake at 350° for 1-1/2 hours or until the meat is tender. **Yield:** 6 servings.

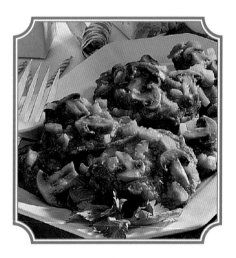

Exchanges: 3-1/2 Lean Meat, 1 Vegetable, 1/2 Fat

Nutritional Information

Serving Size: 1/6 recipe
Calories: 270
Sodium: 107 mg
Cholesterol: 69 mg

Carbohydrate: 11 gm
Protein: 26 gm
Fat: 13 gm
Fiber: 1 gm

Beef and Asparagus Stir-Fry

JoLynn Hill, Roosevelt, Utah

*With tasty tender slices of beef and fresh colorful vegetables,
this mouth-watering stir-fry was designated "a keeper" by my husband the
first time I made it. I appreciate how quick it is to prepare.*

2 tablespoons cornstarch
2 tablespoons plus 1/2 cup water,
 divided
1/2 teaspoon salt-free seasoning
 blend
1/4 teaspoon pepper
1/8 teaspoon hot pepper sauce
1 pound boneless round steak
 (3/4 inch thick)
2 tablespoons vegetable oil,
 divided
2 cups fresh asparagus pieces
1 cup sliced cauliflower
1 small sweet red *or* green
 pepper, julienned
1 small onion, cut into 1/4-inch
 wedges
2 teaspoons low-sodium beef
 bouillon granules
1 tablespoon light soy sauce
1 tablespoon ketchup

1 teaspoon cider *or* red
 wine vinegar
3 cups hot cooked rice

Combine cornstarch, 2 tablespoons water, seasoning blend, pepper and hot pepper sauce. Slice beef into thin 3-in. strips; toss with the cornstarch mixture. In a large skillet or wok over medium-high heat, stir-fry half of the beef in 1 tablespoon oil until cooked as desired; remove from the skillet. Repeat with remaining beef and 1 tablespoon oil. Stir-fry the asparagus and cauliflower for 4 minutes. Add red pepper and onion; stir-fry for 2 minutes. Return beef to skillet. Combine the bouillon, soy sauce, ketchup, vinegar and remaining water; add to the skillet. Bring to a boil. Cook and stir for 2 minutes. Serve over rice. **Yield:** 6 servings.

Exchanges: 2-1/2 Lean Meat, 1-1/2 Starch, 1 Vegetable

Nutritional Information

Serving Size: 1/6 recipe
Calories: 330
Sodium: 250 mg
Cholesterol: 46 mg

Carbohydrate: 32 gm
Protein: 22 gm
Fat: 12 gm
Fiber: 2 gm

Southwestern Stew

Linda Russell, Forest Lakes, Arizona

Here's a savory stew you can make ahead and serve when in a hurry.

2 pounds lean beef stew meat, cut into 1-inch cubes
2 tablespoons vegetable oil
2 cups water
1-1/4 cups chopped onions
1 cup salsa
2 garlic cloves, minced
1 tablespoon dried parsley flakes
2 teaspoons low-sodium beef bouillon granules
1 teaspoon ground cumin
1/2 teaspoon salt-free seasoning blend
5 medium carrots, cut into 1-inch pieces
1 can (14-1/2 ounces) no-salt-added tomatoes, undrained and cut up
2 cups frozen cut green beans
1-1/2 cups frozen corn
1 can (4 ounces) chopped green chilies
1/8 teaspoon hot pepper sauce

In a 4-qt. Dutch oven over medium heat, brown meat in oil; drain. Add the next eight ingredients; bring to a boil. Reduce heat; cover and simmer for 1 hour. Add carrots; return to a boil. Reduce heat and simmer for 20 minutes. Add tomatoes, beans, corn and chilies; return to a boil. Reduce heat; cover and simmer for 15-20 minutes or until beef and vegetables are tender. Season with hot pepper sauce. **Yield:** 10 servings.

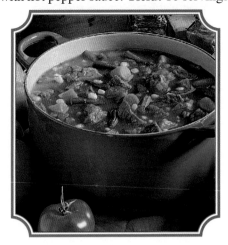

Exchanges: 4 Lean Meat, 2 Vegetable, 1/2 Fat

Nutritional Information

Serving Size: 1/10 recipe
Calories: 321
Sodium: 469 mg
Cholesterol: 92 mg

Carbohydrate: 18 gm
Protein: 32 gm
Fat: 14 gm
Fiber: 4 gm

Beef 'n' Braised Onion Sandwiches

Lois McAtee, Oceanside, California

*These easy sandwiches have been a favorite with our
four grown children since they were teenagers.
They're wonderfully delicious and perfect for any occasion.*

2 tablespoons water
2 teaspoons prepared horseradish
2 teaspoons vegetable oil
2 teaspoons cider *or* red
   wine vinegar
1 cup thinly sliced onion rings
4 hamburger buns *or* onion rolls,
   split
3/4 pound thinly sliced roast beef
4 slices (1 ounce *each*)
   fat-free Monterey Jack cheese

In a skillet over medium heat, combine water, horseradish, oil and vinegar. Add onions; cook and stir until liquid is absorbed and onions are golden, about 12-14 minutes. Place bottom halves of rolls on a baking sheet; top with beef, onion mixture and cheese. Broil 4 in. from the heat for 1-2 minutes or until cheese is melted. Replace roll tops. **Yield:** 4 servings.

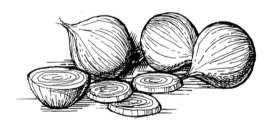

Exchanges: 4 Lean Meat, 1-1/2 Starch, 1 Vegetable, 1/2 Fat

Nutritional Information

Serving Size: 1 sandwich
Calories: 375
Sodium: 916 mg
Cholesterol: 68 mg

Carbohydrate: 30 gm
Protein: 35 gm
Fat: 12 gm
Fiber: 2 gm

Stroganoff Sandwich

Gretchen Kuipers, Platte, South Dakota

I often serve this sandwich to my husband as a hearty main dish when he comes in from working in the field late in the afternoon.

1 **pound lean ground beef**
1/4 **cup chopped onion**
1/4 **teaspoon garlic powder**
Pepper to taste
1 **teaspoon Worcestershire sauce**
1 **can (4 ounces) sliced mushrooms, drained**
1 **cup (8 ounces) light sour cream**
1 **loaf (1 pound) French bread, cut in half lengthwise**
2 **medium tomatoes, thinly sliced**
1 **medium green pepper, cut into rings**
1 **cup (4 ounces) shredded reduced-fat cheddar cheese**

In a skillet, brown beef with onion. Drain. Season with the garlic powder, pepper and Worcestershire sauce. Remove from the heat and stir in mushrooms and sour cream; set aside. Place bread, cut side up, on a baking sheet; broil until light golden brown. Reset oven to 375°. Spread bread with ground beef mixture. Top with the tomatoes, pepper rings and cheese. Bake for 5 minutes or until the cheese melts. Serve immediately. **Yield:** 8 servings.

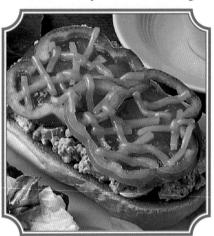

Exchanges: 2 Starch, 2 Lean Meat, 1 Fat, 1/2 Vegetable

Nutritional Information

Serving Size: 1/8 recipe
Calories: 329
Sodium: 562 mg
Cholesterol: 33 mg

Carbohydrate: 35 gm
Protein: 23 gm
Fat: 10 gm
Fiber: 3 gm

Mulligan Stew

Beth Schlea, Gibsonburg, Ohio

This hearty stew is packed with a colorful combination of vegetables and tender pieces of beef.

1/4 cup all-purpose flour
1 teaspoon pepper
1 pound lean beef stew meat, cut into 1-inch cubes
1 tablespoon vegetable oil
2 cans (10-1/2 ounces *each*) low-sodium beef broth
1 cup water
2 bay leaves
1/2 teaspoon garlic powder
1/2 teaspoon dried oregano
1/2 teaspoon dried basil
1/2 teaspoon dill weed
3 medium carrots, cut into 1-inch slices
2 medium potatoes, peeled and cubed
2 celery ribs, cut into 1-inch slices
1 onion, cut into eight wedges
1 cup *each* frozen corn, green beans, lima beans and peas
1 tablespoon cornstarch
2 tablespoons cold water
1 tablespoon minced fresh parsley

Combine flour and pepper; toss with beef cubes. In a Dutch oven, brown beef in oil. Add broth, water, bay leaves, garlic powder, oregano, basil and dill; bring to a boil. Reduce heat; cover and simmer until meat is tender, about 2 hours. Add carrots, potatoes, celery and onion; cover and simmer for 40 minutes. Add corn, beans and peas; cover and simmer 15 minutes longer or until vegetables are tender. Combine cornstarch and cold water until smooth; add to stew. Bring to a boil; cook and stir for 2 minutes. Discard bay leaves; add parsley. **Yield:** 8 servings.

Exchanges: 2-1/2 Lean Meat, 1 Starch, 1 Vegetable

Nutritional Information

Serving Size: 1 cup
Calories: 288
Sodium: 241 mg
Cholesterol: 57 mg
Carbohydrate: 29 gm
Protein: 25 gm
Fat: 9 gm
Fiber: 6 gm

Savory Beef Stew

Kay Fortier, Wildrose, North Dakota

*You'll be surprised at the unique flavor in this stew.
The secret ingredient is cranberry juice.*

1/2 cup all-purpose flour
1 teaspoon salt-free seasoning blend
2 pounds lean beef stew meat,
   cut into 1-inch cubes
4 turkey bacon strips, cut into
   1-inch pieces
10 small onions
2 cups light cranberry juice,
   divided
1 can (14-1/2 ounces) low-sodium
   beef broth
4 whole cloves
1 bay leaf
1/2 teaspoon pepper
1/2 teaspoon dried marjoram
1/4 teaspoon dried thyme
1/4 teaspoon garlic powder
5 medium carrots, cut into
   chunks
5 medium potatoes, peeled and
   cubed
2 cups frozen peas, thawed

In a medium bowl, combine flour and seasoning blend; set aside 2 tablespoons. Add beef to bowl and toss to coat. In a Dutch oven, combine beef and bacon. Bake, uncovered, at 400° for 30 minutes. Add onions, 1-1/2 cups cranberry juice, broth and seasonings. Cover and bake at 350° for 1 hour. Add carrots and potatoes; bake 1 hour or until meat and vegetables are tender. Combine reserved flour mixture and remaining cranberry juice until smooth; stir into stew. Cover and bake 30 minutes longer. Discard bay leaf. Add peas; return to the oven for 5 minutes. **Yield:** 10 servings.

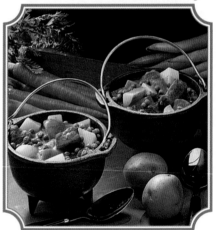

Exchanges: 4 Lean Meat, 2-1/2 Vegetable, 1 Starch

Nutritional Information

Serving Size: 1 cup	Carbohydrate: 38 gm
Calories: 397	Protein: 36 gm
Sodium: 416 mg	Fat: 12 gm
Cholesterol: 97 mg	Fiber: 5 gm

Beef Burritos

Amy Martin, Waddell, Arizona

Living in Arizona, we enjoy all sorts of foods with Southwestern flair, such as these beef-stuffed tortillas. The recipe is easy to make and easy to serve.

2 chuck pot roasts (2-1/2 to 3 pounds *each*)
2 tablespoons vegetable oil
1 cup water
1 large onion, chopped
4 garlic cloves, minced
2 teaspoons dried oregano
2 teaspoons salt-free seasoning blend
1 teaspoon pepper
2 cans (14-1/2 ounces *each*) no-salt-added tomatoes, undrained and cut up
2 cans (4 ounces *each*) chopped green chilies
2 tablespoons all-purpose flour
1/4 cup cold water
4 to 6 drops hot pepper sauce
18 flour tortillas (8 inches), warmed

1 cup plus 2 tablespoons *each* shredded fat-free cheddar cheese, nonfat sour cream and salsa

In a Dutch oven over medium heat, brown roasts in oil; drain. Add water, onion, garlic, oregano, seasoning blend and pepper; bring to a boil. Reduce heat; cover and simmer for 2 to 2-1/2 hours or until meat is tender. Remove roasts; cool. Remove meat from bone and cut into bite-size pieces. Skim fat from pan juices. Add tomatoes and chilies; mix well. Add meat; bring to a boil. Reduce heat; simmer, uncovered, for 30 minutes. Combine flour and cold water until smooth. Stir into beef mixture. Bring to a boil. Cook and stir for 2 minutes or until thickened. Add hot pepper sauce. Spoon down the center of tortillas; fold top and bottom of tortilla over filling and roll up. Serve with cheese, sour cream and salsa. **Yield:** 18 servings.

Exchanges: 2-1/2 Lean Meat, 2 Starch, 1 Vegetable, 1/2 Fat

Nutritional Information

Serving Size: 1/18 recipe
Calories: 351
Sodium: 525 mg
Cholesterol: 66 mg

Carbohydrate: 35 gm
Protein: 30 gm
Fat: 10 gm
Fiber: 2 gm

Spaghetti Pie

Ruth Andrewson, Leavenworth, Washington

*Here's a nice change of pace from traditional spaghetti.
The noodle crust makes a pretty presentation.*

6 ounces spaghetti
Egg substitute equivalent to 2 eggs
1/2 cup grated Parmesan cheese
1 cup low-fat cottage cheese
1 pound lean ground beef
1/2 cup chopped onion
1/4 cup chopped sweet red pepper
1 cup canned no-salt-added whole tomatoes, undrained and cut up
1 can (6 ounces) no-salt-added tomato paste
1 teaspoon sugar
1 teaspoon dried oregano
1/2 teaspoon garlic powder
1/2 cup shredded reduced-fat mozzarella cheese

Cook spaghetti according to package directions; drain and place in a bowl. Add egg substitute and Parmesan cheese; mix well. Spread over the bottom and up the sides of a greased 10-in. deep-dish pie plate. Spoon cottage cheese into crust; set aside. In a skillet, cook beef, onion and red pepper over medium heat until meat is no longer pink; drain. Stir in tomatoes, tomato paste, sugar, oregano and garlic powder. Spoon over cottage cheese. Bake, uncovered, at 350° for 20 minutes. Sprinkle with mozzarella cheese; return to the oven for 5 minutes or until cheese is melted. Cut into wedges. **Yield:** 6 servings.

Exchanges: 4 Lean Meat, 2 Vegetable, 1 Starch, 1 Fat

Nutritional Information

Serving Size: 1/6 recipe
Calories: 398
Sodium: 507 mg
Cholesterol: 43 mg

Carbohydrate: 35 gm
Protein: 35 gm
Fat: 13 gm
Fiber: 3 gm

Tomato Pepper Steak

Carolyn Butterfield, Atkinson, Nebraska

This popular beef dish is tasty as well as colorful.

1 pound round steak, cut into
  1/4-inch x 2-inch strips
1 tablespoon paprika
2 tablespoons reduced-fat
  margarine
1 can (10-1/2 ounces) low-sodium
  beef broth
1 teaspoon low-sodium beef
  bouillon granules
2 garlic cloves, minced
2 medium green peppers, cut into
  strips
1 cup thinly sliced onion
2 tablespoons cornstarch
2 tablespoons light soy sauce
1/3 cup cold water
2 fresh tomatoes, peeled and cut
  into wedges
3 cups cooked rice

Sprinkle meat with paprika. In a large nonstick skillet, melt margarine over medium-high heat. Brown beef. Add broth, bouillon and garlic. Simmer, covered, for 30 minutes. Add green peppers and onion. Cover and continue to simmer for 5 minutes. Combine cornstarch, soy sauce and water until smooth; stir into meat mixture. Bring to a boil. Cook and stir for 2 minutes or until thickened. Gently stir in tomatoes and heat through. Serve over rice. **Yield:** 6 servings.

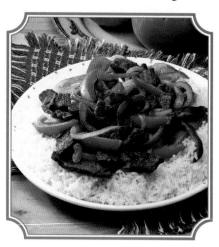

Exchanges: 2-1/2 Lean Meat, 1-1/2 Vegetable, 1-1/2 Starch, 1/2 Fat

Nutritional Information

Serving Size: 1/6 recipe
Calories: 317
Sodium: 405 mg
Cholesterol: 46 mg

Carbohydrate: 35 gm
Protein: 21 gm
Fat: 10 gm
Fiber: 2 gm

Asparagus Shepherd's Pie

Steve Rowland, Fredericksburg, Virginia

Shepherd's pie takes a tasty twist with this version. Between the fluffy mashed potato topping and the savory ground beef base is a bed of tender asparagus. Even my kids ask for big helpings.

6 medium potatoes, peeled and quartered
1 pound lean ground beef
1 large onion, chopped
2 garlic cloves, minced
1 can (10-3/4 ounces) condensed cream of asparagus soup, undiluted
1/4 teaspoon pepper
1 pound fresh asparagus, trimmed and cut into 1-inch pieces
1/2 cup skim milk
2 tablespoons reduced-fat margarine
1 teaspoon rubbed sage
1/2 cup shredded reduced-fat mozzarella cheese
Paprika

In a saucepan, cover potatoes with water; cook until very tender. Meanwhile, in a skillet, cook beef, onion and garlic over medium heat until no longer pink; drain. Stir in soup and pepper; pour into a 2-qt. baking dish coated with nonstick cooking spray. Cook asparagus in a small amount of water until crisp-tender, about 3-4 minutes; drain and place over beef mixture. Drain potatoes; mash with milk, margarine, and sage. Spread over the asparagus. Sprinkle with cheese and paprika. Bake, uncovered, at 350° for 20 minutes. **Yield:** 8 servings.

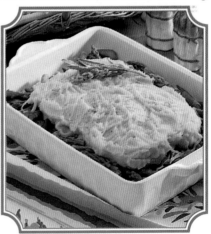

Exchanges: 2 Lean Meat, 1-1/2 Starch, 1 Vegetable, 1/2 Fat

Nutritional Information

Serving Size: 1/8 recipe
Calories: 264
Sodium: 436 mg
Cholesterol: 26 mg

Carbohydrate: 29 gm
Protein: 20 gm
Fat: 10 gm
Fiber: 3 gm

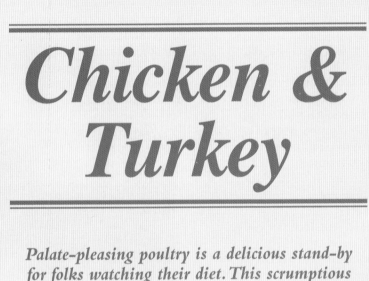

Chicken & Turkey

Palate-pleasing poultry is a delicious stand-by for folks watching their diet. This scrumptious assortment will liven up your recipe collection.

Chicken Mushroom Stew

Kim Marie Van Rheenen, Mendota, Illinois

The flavors blend beautifully in this pot of chicken, vegetables and herbs as it simmers slowly in a slow cooker. Folks with busy schedules will love this convenient recipe.

1-1/2 pounds boneless skinless chicken breasts
2 tablespoons vegetable oil, *divided*
1/2 pound fresh mushrooms, sliced
1 medium onion, diced
3 cups diced zucchini
1 cup diced green pepper
4 garlic cloves, minced
3 medium tomatoes, diced
1 can (6 ounces) no-salt-added tomato paste
3/4 cup water
1 teaspoon salt-free seasoning blend
1 teaspoon *each* dried thyme, oregano, marjoram and basil

Cut chicken into 1-in. cubes; brown in 1 tablespoon oil in a large skillet. Transfer to a slow cooker. In the same skillet, saute the mushrooms, onion, zucchini, green pepper and garlic in remaining oil until crisp-tender. Place in slow cooker. Add tomatoes, tomato paste, water and seasonings. Cover and cook on low for 4 hours or until the vegetables are tender. **Yield:** 6 servings.

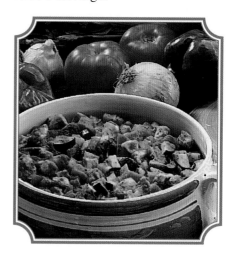

Exchanges: 3-1/2 Lean Meat, 2 Vegetable, 1 Fat

Nutritional Information

Serving Size: 1/6 recipe
Calories: 239
Sodium: 109 mg
Cholesterol: 66 mg

Carbohydrate: 17 gm
Protein: 30 gm
Fat: 7 gm
Fiber: 4 gm

Grilled Turkey Tenderloin

Denise Nebel, Wayland, Iowa

Guests who try my grilled specialty agree the turkey melts in your mouth and the flavor is fantastic.

1/4 cup light soy sauce
1/4 cup vegetable oil
1/4 cup unsweetened apple juice
2 tablespoons lemon juice
2 tablespoons dried minced onion
1 teaspoon vanilla extract
1/4 teaspoon ground ginger
Dash *each* garlic powder and pepper
2 turkey breast tenderloins (1/2 pound *each*)

In a large resealable plastic bag or shallow glass dish, combine the soy sauce, oil, apple juice, lemon juice, onion, vanilla, ginger, garlic powder and pepper. Add turkey; seal or cover and refrigerate for at least 2 hours. Discard marinade. Grill turkey, covered, over medium heat for 8-10 minutes per side or until juices run clear. **Yield:** 4 servings.

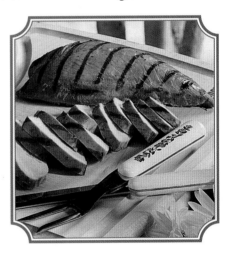

Exchanges: 3-1/2 Lean Meat, 2 Fat

Nutritional Information

Serving Size: 1/4 recipe
Calories: 252
Sodium: 518 mg
Cholesterol: 74 mg

Carbohydrate: 3 gm
Protein: 25 gm
Fat: 15 gm
Fiber: trace

Lemon Herb Chicken

Janice Smith, Cynthiana, Kentucky

This recipe proves that some simple seasonings can really enhance the naturally terrific taste of chicken. I depend on this recipe often in summer.

1/2 cup lemon juice
1/4 cup vegetable oil
1/4 cup minced fresh parsley
1 teaspoon dried tarragon
1/4 teaspoon pepper
8 boneless skinless chicken breast halves (2 pounds)

In a large resealable plastic bag or shallow glass dish, combine the first five ingredients. Add chicken. Seal or cover and refrigerate for 4 hours or overnight. Drain; discard marinade. Grill chicken, uncovered, over medium-low heat for 10-15 minutes or until juices run clear, turning several times. **Yield:** 8 servings.

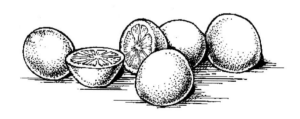

Exchanges: 3-1/2 Lean Meat, 1 Fat

Nutritional Information

Serving Size: 1/8 recipe
Calories: 188
Sodium: 78 mg
Cholesterol: 66 mg

Carbohydrate: 1 gm
Protein: 26 gm
Fat: 8 gm
Fiber: trace

Chicken Stir-Fry

Lori Schlecht, Wimbledon, North Dakota

*This is a tasty, healthy meal that everyone in my house enjoys.
Ginger complements the chicken and vegetables.*

**1 pound boneless skinless chicken
   breasts**
3 tablespoons cornstarch
2 tablespoons light soy sauce
1/2 teaspoon ground ginger
1/4 teaspoon garlic powder
**3 tablespoons vegetable oil,
   *divided***
2 cups broccoli florets
**1 cup sliced celery (1/2-inch
   pieces)**
1 cup thinly sliced carrots
1 small onion, cut into wedges
1 cup water
**1 teaspoon low-sodium chicken
   bouillon granules**
2 cups hot cooked rice

Cut chicken into 1/2-in. strips; place in a resealable plastic bag. Add cornstarch and toss to coat. Combine soy sauce, ginger and garlic powder; add to bag and shake well. Refrigerate for 30 minutes. In a large skillet or wok, heat 2 tablespoons of oil; stir-fry chicken until no longer pink, about 3-5 minutes. Remove and keep warm. Add remaining oil; stir-fry broccoli, celery, carrots and onion for 4-5 minutes or until crisp-tender. Add water and bouillon. Return chicken to pan. Cook and stir until thickened and bubbly. Serve over rice. **Yield:** 4 servings.

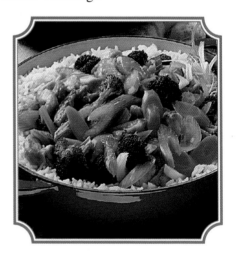

Exchanges: 3-1/2 Lean Meat, 2 Starch, 1 Fat
Nutritional Information
Serving Size: 1/4 recipe
Calories: 394
Sodium: 602 mg
Cholesterol: 67 mg

Carbohydrate: 38 gm
Protein: 31 gm
Fat: 12 gm
Fiber: 3 gm

Parmesan Chicken

Cara Flora, Kokomo, Indiana

*This chicken is moist and saucy with
great Parmesan flavor. It's popular at potlucks.*

**8 boneless skinless chicken
    breast halves (2 pounds)
1 cup fat-free mayonnaise
1/2 cup grated Parmesan cheese
2 teaspoons dried oregano
1/8 teaspoon pepper
Paprika, optional**

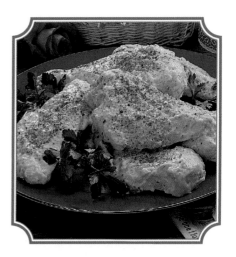

Place chicken in a shallow 3-qt. baking
dish coated with nonstick cooking spray.
Bake, uncovered, at 400° for 20 minutes.
Combine mayonnaise, cheese, oregano
and pepper; spread over chicken. Sprinkle
with paprika if desired. Bake 20 minutes
more or until chicken juices run clear.
Yield: 8 servings.

Exchanges: 4 Lean Meat

Nutritional Information

Serving Size: 1/8 recipe
Calories: 173
Sodium: 400 mg
Cholesterol: 71 mg

Carbohydrate: 4 gm
Protein: 29 gm
Fat: 3 gm
Fiber: 0 gm

Apricot-Glazed Chicken

Lois Collier, Vineland, New Jersey

*My husband has dietary restrictions but still likes good food.
We both agree this slightly sweet chicken is delicious.*

**2 boneless skinless chicken
breast halves (1/2 pound)
1/4 cup apricot spreadable fruit
1-1/2 teaspoons light soy sauce
1 teaspoon Dijon mustard
1 teaspoon honey
1 teaspoon margarine, melted**

Coat a broiler pan with nonstick cooking spray; place chicken on pan. Combine remaining ingredients; brush half over the chicken. Broil 5-6 in. from the heat for 5 minutes. Turn chicken over; brush with remaining apricot mixture. Broil until juices run clear. **Yield:** 2 servings.

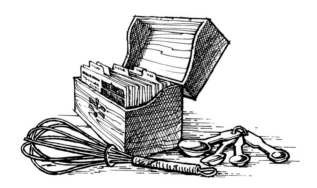

Exchanges: 4 Lean Meat, 1 Fat

Nutritional Information

Serving Size: 1/2 recipe
Calories: 298
Sodium: 307 mg
Cholesterol: 66 mg

Carbohydrate: 3 gm
Protein: 27 gm
Fat: 3 gm
Fiber: trace

Turkey Pasta Primavera

Marilyn Schafer, Weidman, Michigan

This is a fast, easy and satisfying recipe that calls for turkey and a wide array of vegetables. The sauce is a great way to get kids to eat their vegetables.

8 ounces fettuccine *or* spaghetti
1 cup broccoli florets
1 cup julienned carrots
1/2 cup chopped sweet red pepper
2 tablespoons all-purpose flour
1-3/4 cups skim milk
1 package (8 ounces) light cream cheese, cubed
1/2 cup chopped green onions
3/4 teaspoon Italian seasoning
1/4 teaspoon garlic powder
1/8 teaspoon pepper
1/2 teaspoon salt-free seasoning blend
2 cups julienned cooked turkey breast
1/2 cup nonfat Parmesan cheese topping

Cook pasta according to package directions, adding broccoli, carrots and red pepper during the last 5 minutes. Meanwhile, in a medium saucepan, stir flour and milk until smooth. Add the cream cheese, onions and seasonings; bring to a boil over medium-low heat. Cook and stir 1-2 minutes. Add turkey and Parmesan cheese topping; heat through. Drain pasta; toss with cheese sauce. **Yield:** 6 servings.

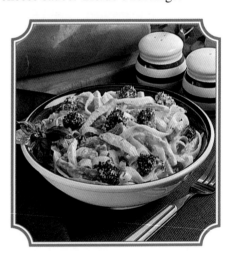

Exchanges: 3-1/2 Lean Meat, 1-1/2 Starch, 1 Vegetable, 1/2 Fat

Nutritional Information

Serving Size: 1/6 recipe
Calories: 369
Sodium: 362 mg
Cholesterol: 79 mg

Carbohydrate: 38 gm
Protein: 42 gm
Fat: 5 gm
Fiber: 3 gm

Chicken Vegetable Medley

Kim Marie Van Rheenen, Mendota, Illinois

Garden-fresh vegetables, herbs and tender chicken combine in this dish. It's a mouth-watering meal sure to earn you raves.

6 boneless skinless chicken breast halves (1-1/2 pounds)
3 tablespoons olive *or* vegetable oil, *divided*
1/2 pound fresh mushrooms, sliced
4 garlic cloves, minced
3 tomatoes, peeled, seeded and chopped
2 medium eggplant, peeled and diced
2 large green peppers, diced
2 medium zucchini, diced
1 large onion, diced
1 can (8 ounces) no-salt-added tomato sauce
1 bay leaf
1 teaspoon dried basil
1 teaspoon dried oregano
1/2 teaspoon dried marjoram
1/2 teaspoon dried thyme
1/2 teaspoon salt-free seasoning blend
1/4 teaspoon pepper

In a Dutch oven over medium heat, brown chicken in 1 tablespoon of oil; set chicken aside. Add remaining oil to Dutch oven; saute mushrooms, garlic, tomatoes, eggplant, green peppers, zucchini and onion for 10-15 minutes or until vegetables are tender. Add remaining ingredients; bring to a boil. Return chicken to pan. Reduce heat; cover and simmer to 15-20 minutes or until chicken juices run clear. Discard bay leaf before serving. **Yield:** 6 servings.

Exchanges: 3-1/2 Lean Meat, 1 Vegetable, 1 Fat, 1/2 Starch

Nutritional Information

Serving Size: 1/6 recipe
Calories: 291
Sodium: 92 mg
Cholesterol: 66 mg

Carbohydrate: 24 gm
Protein: 31 gm
Fat: 9 gm
Fiber: 7 gm

Chicken Creole

Dolly Hall, Wheelwright, Kentucky

If you like dishes with a little zip, this recipe fits the bill.

1-1/2 pounds boneless skinless chicken breasts, cut into 1-inch cubes
1 teaspoon salt-free seasoning blend, *divided*
1/4 teaspoon pepper
1 tablespoon vegetable oil
1 cup finely chopped onion
1/2 cup finely sliced celery
1/2 cup diced green pepper
2 garlic cloves, minced
1 can (14-1/2 ounces) no-salt-added tomatoes, undrained and cut up
1/2 cup plus 1 tablespoon water
1-1/2 teaspoons paprika
1/8 teaspoon cayenne pepper
1 bay leaf
2 teaspoons cornstarch
3 cups hot cooked rice

Combine chicken, 1/2 teaspoon seasoning blend and pepper; toss lightly. In a large skillet over medium heat, brown chicken in oil; remove and set aside. In the same skillet, saute the onion, celery, green pepper and garlic until tender. Stir in tomatoes, 1/2 cup water, paprika, cayenne pepper, bay leaf and remaining seasoning blend; bring to a boil. Reduce heat; cover and simmer for 10 minutes. Add chicken. Combine cornstarch and remaining water until smooth; stir into chicken mixture and bring to a boil. Simmer, uncovered, for 10-15 minutes or until chicken is tender. Discard bay leaf before serving. Serve over rice. **Yield:** 4 servings.

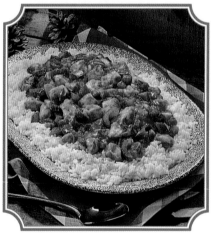

Exchanges: 3-1/2 Lean Meat, , 1-1/2 Vegetable, 1 Starch

Nutritional Information

Serving Size: 1/6 recipe
Calories: 287
Sodium: 100 mg
Cholesterol: 66 mg

Carbohydrate: 32 gm
Protein: 30 gm
Fat: 4 gm
Fiber: 2 gm

Autumn Chicken

Debbi Jo Mullins, Canoga Park, California

*Although my husband typically favors rich foods, he delights in eating
this light sweet chicken. Apples and chicken are perfect partners.*

1 large onion, sliced
1 tablespoon olive *or* vegetable oil
2 cups sliced peeled tart apples
**6 boneless skinless chicken
    breast halves (1-1/2 pounds)**
1-1/2 cups unsweetened apple juice
2 tablespoons honey

In a nonstick skillet, saute onion in oil until tender; add apples and saute 1 minute longer. Place chicken in a 13-in. x 9-in. x 2-in. baking dish coated with nonstick cooking spray. Top with onion mixture. Combine apple juice and honey; pour over all. Cover and bake at 350° for 45 minutes or until chicken juices run clear. **Yield:** 6 servings.

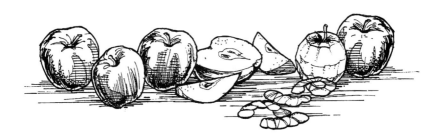

Exchanges: 3-1/2 Lean Meat, 1 Fruit, 1/2 Vegetable, 1/2 Fat

Nutritional Information

Serving Size: 1/6 recipe
Calories: 231
Sodium: 77 mg
Cholesterol: 66 mg

Carbohydrate: 22 gm
Protein: 27 gm
Fat: 4 gm
Fiber: 1 gm

Chicken and Tomato Scampi

Jan Gridley, Elverson, Pennsylvania

My mother had a knack for turning ordinary ingredients into "lively" meals. I try to do the same, but nothing can compare to Mom's cooking!

2 to 3 garlic cloves, minced
1/4 cup chopped green onions
2 tablespoons reduced-fat margarine
1 tablespoon olive *or* vegetable oil
1 pound boneless skinless chicken breasts, cut into 1-inch pieces
1 teaspoon salt-free seasoning blend
1/2 teaspoon pepper
1 can (14-1/2 ounces) Italian stewed tomatoes
1/4 cup lemon juice
1/2 teaspoon sugar
2 teaspoons cornstarch
2 teaspoons cold water
1/4 cup chopped fresh parsley
2 cups hot cooked rice

In a nonstick skillet over medium heat, saute garlic and onions in margarine and oil until onions are tender. Add chicken, seasoning blend and pepper. Cook for 6-8 minutes or until chicken juices run clear. Add tomatoes, lemon juice and sugar; heat through. Combine cornstarch and water until smooth; stir into chicken mixture. Bring to a boil; cook and stir for 2 minutes or until thickened. Add parsley. Serve over rice. **Yield:** 4 servings.

Exchanges: 3-1/2 Lean Meat, 1-1/2 Vegetable, 1 Starch, 1 Fat

Nutritional Information

Serving Size: 1/4 recipe
Calories: 338
Sodium: 365 mg
Cholesterol: 66 mg

Carbohydrate: 33 gm
Protein: 29 gm
Fat: 9 gm
Fiber: 2 gm

Cool Cucumber Chicken

Andria Barosi-Stampone, Randolph, New Jersey

*My husband really likes chicken and is especially fond of this recipe.
It's versatile because it can be served hot or cold.*

**4 boneless skinless chicken breast
halves (1 pound)**
**2 tablespoons olive *or*
vegetable oil**
**1 medium cucumber, seeded and
chopped**
1/2 cup plain low-fat yogurt
**2 tablespoons reduced-fat
mayonnaise**
1 tablespoon minced fresh dill
1/8 teaspoon pepper

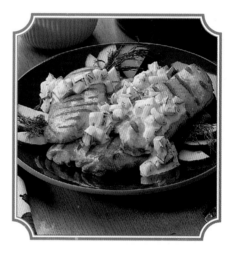

Brush both sides of chicken with oil. Broil 5 in. from the heat or grill over medium heat, turning occasionally, for 10-14 minutes or until juices run clear. Meanwhile, combine remaining ingredients in a small bowl. Spoon over warm chicken; serve immediately. Or, to serve cold, spoon sauce over chicken and refrigerate several hours or overnight. **Yield:** 4 servings.

Exchanges: 3-1/2 Lean Meat, 1/2 Fat
Nutritional Information
Serving Size: 1/4 recipe
Calories: 222
Sodium: 166 mg
Cholesterol: 68 mg

Carbohydrate: 5 gm
Protein: 28 gm
Fat: 9 gm
Fiber: trace

Harvest Chicken

Linda Hutton, Hayden, Idaho

This chicken has become a Sunday–dinner standby around our house. Friends and family comment on the fresh combination of asparagus, carrots, potatoes and chicken.

1/3 **cup all-purpose flour**
1/4 **teaspoon paprika**
  4 **boneless skinless chicken breast halves (1 pound)**
  1 **tablespoon vegetable oil**
  2 **cups low-sodium chicken broth,** *divided*
  1 **teaspoon dill weed**
3/4 **teaspoon salt-free seasoning blend**
1/4 **teaspoon dried basil**
1/4 **teaspoon pepper**
  4 **medium potatoes, cut into bite-size pieces**
  3 **medium carrots, cut into 2-inch pieces**
1/2 **pound fresh asparagus, cut into 2-inch pieces**
  2 **tablespoons snipped fresh parsley**

Combine the flour and paprika; set aside 2 tablespoons. Coat chicken in remaining mixture. In a nonstick skillet, brown chicken in oil over medium heat. Drain and set chicken aside. Combine 3/4 cup broth, dill, seasoning blend, basil and pepper in the same skillet; bring to a boil. Add potatoes and carrots. Reduce heat; cover and simmer for 10 minutes. Add chicken; cook for 10 minutes. Add asparagus; cook 15-20 minutes or until chicken juices run clear and vegetables are tender. Combine reserved flour mixture and remaining broth until smooth; stir into skillet. Bring to a boil; cook and stir for 2 minutes or until slightly thickened. Sprinkle with parsley. **Yield:** 4 servings.

Exchanges: 3-1/2 Lean Meat, 1-1/2 Vegetable, 1-1/2 Starch, 1/2 Fat

Nutritional Information

Serving Size: 1/4 recipe
Calories: 348
Sodium: 163 mg
Cholesterol: 68 mg

Carbohydrate: 43 gm
Protein: 35 gm
Fat: 6 gm
Fiber: 5 gm

Turkey Sausage Saute

Susan Lynn Hauser, Etters, Pennsylvania

A good friend gave me this recipe years ago. Since then, I've made it for weekday dinners, special occasions and potlucks. It always disappears quickly.

4 medium potatoes (about 1-1/2 pounds), peeled and cut into 1-inch pieces
1 pound Italian turkey sausage, cut into 1-inch pieces
2 cups cubed skinless turkey breast
1 *each* large green pepper, sweet red pepper and onion, cut into 1-inch pieces
1 package (10 ounces) frozen green beans, thawed
1/2 cup water
1 teaspoon dried oregano
3/4 teaspoon salt-free seasoning blend
1/4 teaspoon pepper

In a large nonstick skillet over medium heat, brown potatoes and sausage for 15-20 minutes. Add turkey, peppers and onion; saute for 15 minutes or until turkey is browned. Add beans, water, oregano, seasoning blend and pepper. Reduce heat; cover and simmer for 15 minutes or until vegetables are tender. **Yield:** 6 servings.

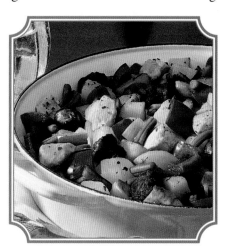

Exchanges: 3-1/2 Lean Meat, 2 Vegetable, 1 Bread

Nutritional Information

Serving Size: 1/6 recipe
Calories: 306
Sodium: 705 mg
Cholesterol: 89 mg

Carbohydrate: 32 gm
Protein: 31 gm
Fat: 8 gm
Fiber: 5 gm

Honey-Citrus Chicken Sandwiches

Claire Batherson, Westchester, Illinois

During the summer months, our kids keep me busy. So it's a welcome relief when my husband volunteers to cook out. This is his specialty.

6 **boneless skinless chicken breast halves (1-1/2 pounds)**
1/4 **cup unsweetened orange juice**
1/4 **cup lemon juice**
1/4 **cup honey**
2 **tablespoons vegetable oil**
1 **tablespoon yellow mustard**
1/4 **teaspoon poultry seasoning**
1/8 **to 1/4 teaspoon cayenne pepper**
6 **slices reduced-fat Monterey Jack cheese (1 ounce *each*)**
6 **kaiser rolls, split**
6 **thin tomato slices**
6 **red onion slices**
Shredded lettuce

Pound chicken breasts until uniform in thickness; set aside. In a large resealable plastic bag or glass 13-in. x 9-in. x 2-in. baking dish, combine orange and lemon juices, honey, oil, mustard, poultry seasoning and cayenne pepper. Add chicken; turn to coat. Close bag or cover and refrigerate for 6-8 hours. Drain, discarding marinade. Grill chicken, uncovered, over medium-low heat, turning occasionally, for 10-12 minutes or until juices run clear. Top each chicken breast with a slice of cheese and grill 1-2 minutes longer or until cheese begins to melt. Serve on rolls with tomato, onion and lettuce. **Yield:** 6 servings.

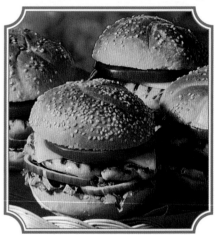

Exchanges: 3-1/2 Lean Meat, 2-1/2 Starch, 1 Fat

Nutritional Information

Serving Size: 1 sandwich	Carbohydrate: 52 gm
Calories: 518	Protein: 43 gm
Sodium: 680 mg	Fat: 16 gm
Cholesterol: 86 mg	Fiber: 3 gm

Zesty Chicken and Rice

Ella West, Lake Charles, Louisiana

A friend gave me this recipe years ago. Italian dressing and seasoning add just the right amount of zip. With chicken, vegetables and rice, it's a meal in one.

6 bone-in chicken breast halves, skin removed
1/3 cup fat-free Italian salad dressing
1 can (14-1/2 ounces) low-sodium chicken broth
1 bag (16 ounces) frozen broccoli, carrots and water chestnuts
2/3 cup uncooked long grain rice
1-1/4 teaspoons Italian seasoning

Place chicken in a greased 13-in. x 9-in. x 2-in. baking dish. Pour dressing over chicken. Bake, uncovered, at 400° for 20 minutes. Combine broth, vegetables, rice and Italian seasoning; pour over chicken. Cover and bake at 350° for 30 minutes. Uncover; bake 30 minutes more or until chicken juices run clear and rice is tender. **Yield:** 6 servings.

SKINNING CHICKEN. To remove the skin from chicken breasts, place chicken skin side up on a cutting board. Grasp the skin at the thickest end of the breast and pull it away. You may want to use paper towel to get a better grip.

Exchanges: 4-1/2 Lean Meat, 1 Starch, 1/2 Vegetable, 1/2 Fat

Nutritional Information

Serving Size: 1/6 recipe
Calories: 363
Sodium: 344 mg
Cholesterol: 94 mg

Carbohydrate: 22 gm
Protein: 34 gm
Fat: 14 gm
Fiber: 3 gm

Taco Skillet Supper

Edna Havens, Wann, Oklahoma

Using ground turkey breast in place of traditional ground beef makes this meal a little lighter, but without sacrificing flavor.

4 cups thinly sliced peeled potatoes
1 small onion, chopped, *divided*
1 teaspoon low-sodium chicken
   bouillon granules
1 cup hot water
1 pound ground turkey breast
1 envelope low-sodium taco
   seasoning mix
1/4 cup skim milk
1-1/4 cups salsa, *divided*
1/2 cup quick-cooking oats
Egg substitute equivalent to 1 egg

Coat a 2-qt. baking dish with nonstick cooking spray; add potatoes and 1 tablespoon onion. Dissolve bouillon in water; pour 1/2 cup over potatoes. Combine turkey, taco seasoning, milk, 1/4 cup salsa, oats, egg substitute and remaining onion; mix well. Spread over potatoes. Combine remaining salsa and chicken broth; pour over the turkey mixture. Bake, uncovered, at 350° for 1 hour or until the potatoes are tender. **Yield:** 8 servings.

> **POTATO POINTERS.** It's easiest to peel potatoes with a vegetable peeler. Be sure to cut away any eyes or green spots as you peel. To keep sliced potatoes from darkening before cooking, keep them immersed in cold water.

Exchanges: 2 Lean Meat, 1 Starch, 1/2 Vegetable
Nutritional Information

Serving Size: 1/8 recipe
Calories: 181
Sodium: 287 mg
Cholesterol: 36 mg

Carbohydrate: 24 gm
Protein: 18 gm
Fat: 1 gm
Fiber: 3 gm

Waldorf Sandwiches

Darlene Sutton, Arvada, Colorado

The fresh fruity filling for this sandwich is a nice variation of a classic. My clan loves the cool and creamy combination, so I serve these sandwiches often for a light lunch or dinner.

1 can (20 ounces) unsweetened crushed pineapple
3 cups cubed cooked turkey breast
1 medium red apple, chopped
1 medium green apple, chopped
1/2 cup chopped walnuts
1 cup sliced celery
1 cup fat-free mayonnaise
1 tablespoon poppy seeds
1 teaspoon grated lemon peel
1/2 teaspoon vanilla extract
1/2 teaspoon salt-free seasoning blend
16 hard rolls, split

Drain pineapple, pressing out excess juice; reserve 1/4 cup juice. In a large bowl, combine pineapple, turkey, apples, walnuts and celery. In a small bowl, combine mayonnaise, poppy seeds, lemon peel, vanilla, seasoning blend and reserved pineapple juice. Pour over turkey mixture and toss well. Chill. Serve on rolls. **Yield:** 16 servings.

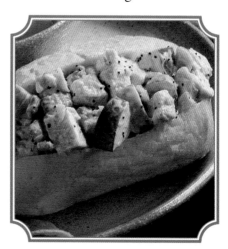

Exchanges: 2-1/2 Starch, 1 Lean Meat, 1 Fat, 1/2 Fruit

Nutritional Information

Serving Size: 1 sandwich
Calories: 314
Sodium: 475 mg
Cholesterol: 22 mg

Carbohydrate: 45 gm
Protein: 16 gm
Fat: 8 gm
Fiber: 3 gm

Turkey Garden Medley

Dohreen Winkler, Howell, Michigan

After you sample this dish, it will quickly become a favorite.

1 pound boneless skinless turkey breast, cut into strips
1 garlic clove, minced
3 tablespoons margarine, *divided*
1 small yellow squash, julienned
1 small zucchini, julienned
1/2 cup *each* julienned green and sweet red pepper
1/4 cup thinly sliced onion
2 tablespoons all-purpose flour
1/2 teaspoon salt-free seasoning blend
1/4 teaspoon pepper
3/4 cup low-sodium chicken broth
1/2 cup evaporated skim milk
8 ounces angel hair pasta, cooked and drained
2 tablespoons shredded Parmesan cheese

In a large nonstick skillet over medium-high heat, saute turkey and garlic in 1 tablespoon margarine for 10-12 minutes or until juices run clear. Add vegetables; cook until crisp-tender. Set aside. In a small saucepan, melt remaining margarine. Add flour, seasoning blend and pepper; stir to form a smooth paste. Gradually add broth, stirring constantly. Bring to a boil; cook for 2 minutes or until thickened. Stir in milk and heat through. Pour over turkey and vegetables; stir until well mixed. Place pasta in a 2-qt. baking dish coated with nonstick cooking spray. Pour turkey mixture over top. Sprinkle with Parmesan cheese. Cover and bake at 350° for 20 minutes; uncover and bake 10 minutes longer. **Yield:** 6 servings.

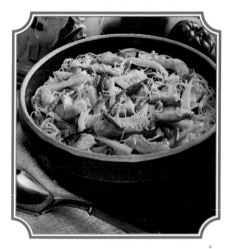

Exchanges: 2-1/2 Lean Meat, 1 Vegetable, 1/2 Starch, 1/2 Fat

Nutritional Information

Serving Size: 1/6 recipe
Calories: 199
Sodium: 227 mg
Cholesterol: 47 mg

Carbohydrate: 14 gm
Protein: 23 gm
Fat: 6 gm
Fiber: 2 gm

30-Minute Chicken

John Kosmas, Minneapolis, Minnesota

*I like to help out in the kitchen whenever I can.
This one-pan meal is great when entertaining because
it can be prepared in a hurry and bakes in no time.*

1 medium onion, sliced
4 boneless skinless chicken breast
  halves (1 pound)
1/2 teaspoon salt-free seasoning
  blend
1/4 teaspoon pepper
1/2 pound fresh mushrooms, sliced
2 medium zucchini, sliced
2 garlic cloves, minced
1 can (14-1/2 ounces) no-salt-added
  tomatoes, undrained and cut up
3/4 teaspoon dried basil
1/2 teaspoon dried oregano
2 tablespoons nonfat Parmesan
  cheese topping

Place onion and chicken in a 13-in. x 9-in. x 2-in. baking dish coated with nonstick cooking spray; sprinkle with seasoning blend and pepper. Layer mushrooms and zucchini over chicken. Combine garlic, tomatoes, basil and oregano; pour over vegetables. Cover tightly. Bake at 450° for 30 minutes or until chicken juices run clear. Sprinkle with Parmesan cheese topping. **Yield:** 4 servings.

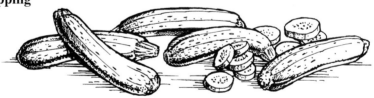

Exchanges: 3 Lean Meat, 2 Vegetable

Nutritional Information

Serving Size: 1/4 recipe
Calories: 184
Sodium: 137 mg
Cholesterol: 66 mg

Carbohydrate: 12 gm
Protein: 30 gm
Fat: 2 gm
Fiber: 2 gm

Chicken Stew

Linda Emery, Tuckerman, Arkansas

Rely on this slow cooker stew on busy weekends when you'd rather not be in the kitchen. Chicken, vegetables and seasonings give this stew great flavor.

2 pounds boneless skinless
   chicken breasts, cut into
   1-inch cubes
2 cans (14-1/2 ounces *each*)
   low-sodium chicken broth
3 cups cubed peeled potatoes
1 cup chopped onion
1 cup sliced celery
1 cup thinly sliced carrots
1 teaspoon paprika
1/2 teaspoon pepper
1/2 teaspoon rubbed sage

1/2 teaspoon dried thyme
1 can (6 ounces) no-salt-added
   tomato paste
1/4 cup cold water
3 tablespoons cornstarch

In a slow cooker, combine the first 11 ingredients; cover and cook on high for 4 hours. Combine water and cornstarch until smooth; stir into stew. Cover and cook 30 minutes more or until the vegetables are tender. **Yield:** 8 servings.

THICKENING WITH CORNSTARCH. Cornstarch easily forms lumps when combined with a warm liquid. So it's important to mix cornstarch with a small amount of cold liquid until smooth before adding it to the hot mixture.

Exchanges: 3-1/2 Lean Meat, 1 Vegetable, 1/2 Starch
Nutritional Information
Serving Size: 1/8 recipe
Calories: 242
Sodium: 173 mg
Cholesterol: 68 mg

Carbohydrate: 24 gm
Protein: 30 gm
Fat: 3 gm
Fiber: 3 gm

Turkey Meat Loaf

Ruby Rath, New Haven, Indiana

I first made this recipe when my husband and I had to start watching our diet. Since then, I've been asked for the recipe many times.

2 pounds ground turkey breast
1 cup quick-cooking oats
1 medium onion, chopped
1/2 cup shredded carrot
1/2 cup skim milk
Egg substitute equivalent to 1 egg
2 tablespoons ketchup
1 teaspoon garlic powder
1/4 teaspoon pepper
TOPPING:
1/4 cup ketchup
1/4 cup quick-cooking oats

In a large bowl, combine the first nine ingredients; mix well. Press into a 9-in. x 5-in. x 3-in. loaf pan coated with nonstick cooking spray. Combine topping ingredients; spread over loaf. Bake, uncovered, at 350° for 65 minutes or until a meat thermometer reads 170° and juices run clear. **Yield:** 10 servings.

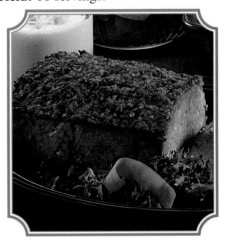

Exchanges: 3 Lean Meat, 1/2 Starch

Nutritional Information

Serving Size: 1/10 recipe
Calories: 167
Sodium: 174 mg
Cholesterol: 57 mg

Carbohydrate: 12 gm
Protein: 26 gm
Fat: 1 gm
Fiber: 2 gm

Chicken and Asparagus

Janet Hill, Sacramento, California

With this recipe, you'll see fancy foods don't necessarily mean a lot of fuss. These "bundles" are prepared in no time and bake in the oven for a quick tasty dinner.

1 pound boneless skinless chicken breasts
24 fresh asparagus spears, trimmed
1/3 cup fat-free Italian salad dressing
2 teaspoons light soy sauce
1/2 teaspoon ground ginger
1/2 teaspoon salt-free seasoning blend
1/8 teaspoon pepper
2 tablespoons sesame seeds
2 cups hot cooked white and wild rice blend

Cut chicken breasts into 1/2-in.-wide strips. Wrap two or three strips around three asparagus spears. Repeat with the remaining chicken and asparagus. Arrange in a 13-in. x 9-in. x 2-in. baking dish coated with nonstick cooking spray. Combine salad dressing, soy sauce, ginger, seasoning blend and pepper. Pour over the chicken bundles. Cover and bake at 350° for 25 minutes. Uncover; sprinkle with sesame seeds and bake 15 minutes longer or until chicken juices run clear. Serve over rice. **Yield:** 4 servings.

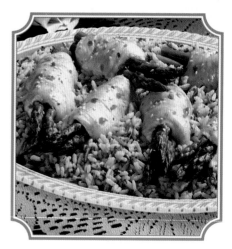

Exchanges: 3-1/2 Lean Meat, 1 Starch

Nutritional Information

Serving Size: 1/4 recipe
Calories: 276
Sodium: 421 mg
Cholesterol: 66 mg

Carbohydrate: 30 gm
Protein: 31 gm
Fat: 3 gm
Fiber: 4 gm

Chicken-Mushroom Loaf

Pearl Altman, Spring Church, Pennsylvania

*Our to-do list of house projects never seems to be complete.
After a hard day's work, it's nice to sit down to this chicken loaf.*

1 can (10-3/4 ounces) reduced-fat, reduced-sodium condensed cream of mushroom soup, undiluted
2/3 cup skim milk
Egg substitute equivalent to 2 eggs
3 cups cubed cooked chicken breast
1 cup cooked rice
1 cup dry bread crumbs
1 jar (2 ounces) diced pimientos, drained
1 teaspoon onion powder
1 teaspoon celery seed
1/2 teaspoon salt-free seasoning blend
1/2 teaspoon paprika
1/4 teaspoon pepper

In a large bowl, combine soup, milk and egg substitute; stir until well mixed. Add all remaining ingredients and mix well. Pour into an 8-in. x 4-in. x 2-in. loaf pan coated with nonstick cooking spray. Bake, uncovered, at 325° for 50-55 minutes. Let stand for 10 minutes before serving. **Yield:** 6 servings.

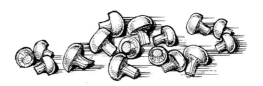

Exchanges: 3 Lean Meat, 1 Starch, 1/2 Vegetable, 1/2 Fat

Nutritional Information

Serving Size: 1/6 recipe
Calories: 274
Sodium: 608 mg
Cholesterol: 62 mg

Carbohydrate: 27 gm
Protein: 28 gm
Fat: 5 gm
Fiber: 1 gm

Chicken and Spinach Supper

Donna Nizolek, Chester, New York

This recipe appeared in a school cookbook I put together while working as a teacher's aide. Everyone will think you fussed all day... but it just takes minutes to put together.

4 packages (10 ounces *each*) frozen chopped spinach, thawed and well drained
1/4 teaspoon ground nutmeg
1 teaspoon salt-free seasoning blend, *divided*
4 cups diced cooked chicken breast
1/4 cup margarine
1/4 cup all-purpose flour
1/4 teaspoon pepper
1/8 teaspoon paprika
2 cups low-sodium chicken broth
1 tablespoon lemon juice
1/2 teaspoon dried rosemary, crushed
TOPPING:
1 tablespoon margarine, melted
1/2 cup dry bread crumbs
1/3 cup nonfat Parmesan cheese topping

Mix spinach, nutmeg and 1/2 teaspoon seasoning blend. Pat in the bottom of a 13-in. x 9-in. x 2-in. baking dish coated with nonstick cooking spray. Top with chicken. Melt margarine in a saucepan. Add flour, pepper, paprika and remaining seasoning blend; stir to form a smooth paste. Gradually add broth, lemon juice and rosemary, stirring constantly. Bring to a boil; cook and stir for 2 minutes or until thickened. Pour over chicken. Combine topping ingredients; sprinkle over casserole. Bake, uncovered, at 350° for 40-45 minutes or until bubbly. **Yield:** 8 servings.

Exchanges: 3 Lean Meat, 1 Vegetable, 1/2 Starch, 1/2 Fat

Nutritional Information

Serving Size: 1/8 recipe
Calories: 265
Sodium: 341 mg
Cholesterol: 64 mg

Carbohydrate: 15 gm
Protein: 29 gm
Fat: 10 gm
Fiber: 5 gm

Red Beans and Sausage

Cathy Webster, Morris, Illinois

Turkey sausage makes this traditional dish deliciously different, while a zesty blend of seasoning adds some spark.

2 garlic cloves, minced
1 medium green pepper, diced
1 medium onion, chopped
1 tablespoon vegetable oil
2 cans (16 ounces *each*) kidney beans, rinsed and drained
1/2 pound reduced-fat smoked turkey sausage, sliced
3/4 cup water
1 teaspoon Cajun seasoning
1/8 teaspoon hot pepper sauce
3 cups hot cooked rice

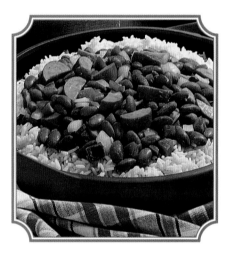

In a saucepan, saute garlic, green pepper and onion in oil until tender, about 5 minutes. Add the next five ingredients; bring to a boil. Reduce heat; cook for 5-7 minutes or until the sausage is heated through. Serve over rice. **Yield:** 6 servings.

Exchanges: 3 Starch, 1 Lean Meat, 1 Fat, 1/2 Vegetable

Nutritional Information

Serving Size: 1/6 recipe
Calories: 377
Sodium: 232 mg
Cholesterol: 31 mg

Carbohydrate: 58 gm
Protein: 20 gm
Fat: 7 gm
Fiber: 14 gm

Easy Baked Chicken

Christine Richburg, Brewton, Alabama

This chicken is a taste treat for those on a special diet.
It turns out so moist.

1 packet (1/2 ounce) butter
  flavored mix*
3/4 cup low-sodium tomato juice
2 tablespoons cider *or* red
  wine vinegar
1 tablespoon light soy sauce
1 teaspoon ground ginger
1 garlic clove, minced
1/2 teaspoon dried oregano
1 broiler/fryer chicken (3 pounds),
  cut up and skin removed

Prepare butter granules according to package directions. Stir in tomato juice, vinegar, soy sauce, ginger, garlic and oregano. Place chicken in a resealable plastic bag. Add marinade; seal and refrigerate for 8 hours or overnight. Place chicken and marinade in a 13-in. x 9-in. x 2-in. baking pan coated with nonstick spray. Bake, uncovered, at 375° for 1 hour or until chicken juices run clear, spooning marinade over chicken several times. **Yield:** 6 servings. ***Editor's Note:** This recipe was tested with Butter Buds butter flavored mix.

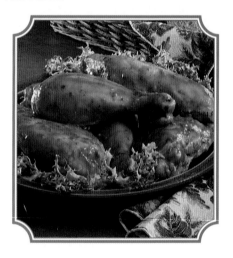

Exchanges: 2-1/2 Lean Meat, 1-1/2 Fat

Nutritional Information

Serving Size: 1/6 recipe
Calories: 192
Sodium: 178 mg
Cholesterol: 64 mg

Carbohydrate: 2 gm
Protein: 16 gm
Fat: 13 gm
Fiber: trace

Grilled Curry Chicken

Schelby Thompson, Dover, Delaware

*We're fortunate to have mild winters, so we
fire up the grill throughout the year. Of all the dishes I prepare,
my family enjoys this slightly spicy chicken the most.*

1 **broiler/fryer chicken (3 pounds),
    cut up and skin removed**
1 **carton (8 ounces) plain nonfat
    yogurt**
1 **medium onion, quartered**
2 **garlic cloves**
2 **tablespoons curry powder**
1 **tablespoon paprika**
1-1/2 **teaspoons salt-free seasoning
    blend**
1/4 **teaspoon cayenne pepper**

Pierce chicken liberally with a fork, then make 1/2-in.- deep diagonal cuts, about 1 in. apart, in the meat. Place in a large re-sealable plastic bag or a glass 13-in. x 9-in. x 2-in. baking dish; set aside. In a blender or food processor, combine yogurt, onion, garlic, curry, paprika, seasoning blend and cayenne pepper; cover and process until smooth. Reserve 1/4 cup for basting; cover and refrigerate. Pour remaining mixture over chicken; turn to coat. Close bag or cover and refrigerate for at least 8 hours. Drain, discarding marinade. Grill chicken, covered, over medium heat, turning and basting with reserved yogurt mixture every 5 minutes, for 30-40 minutes or until juices run clear. **Yield:** 4 servings.

CURRY POWDER CAUTION. If you're not sure how your family will like the flavor of curry powder, use less than what's called for in a recipe, taste the cooked dish and then gradually add more if desired.

Exchanges: 3 Lean Meat, 1-1/2 Fat, 1/2 Vegetable, 1/2 Skim Milk

Nutritional Information

Serving Size: 1/4 recipe
Calories: 295
Sodium: 128 mg
Cholesterol: 86 mg

Carbohydrate: 9 gm
Protein: 25 gm
Fat: 17 gm
Fiber: 1 gm

Herbed Chicken

Diane Cigel, Stevens Point, Wisconsin

This is such a versatile dish because it can be made in the oven or microwave...so time is never a factor. People always comment on the chicken's wonderful subtle herb flavor.

1 cup boiling water
1 tablespoon low-sodium chicken bouillon granules
1/2 teaspoon dried thyme
1/2 teaspoon dried rosemary, crushed
2 bay leaves
1 broiler/fryer chicken (3 pounds)
1 pound new potatoes, halved
2 medium onions, cut into 1/2-inch pieces
2 carrots, cut into 1/2-inch pieces

Combine water, bouillon, thyme, rosemary and bay leaves; pour into a roasting pan. Add chicken; arrange the potatoes, onions and carrots around it. Cover and bake at 350° for 50 minutes. Uncover; bake for 20-30 minutes or until vegetables are tender and chicken juices run clear. Discard the bay leaves and chicken skin before serving. **Yield:** 4 servings.

GET TO KNOW NEW POTATOES! New potatoes have a crisp, waxy texture and thin skins, making them excellent for roasting and boiling. Store new potatoes in a cool, dry, well-ventilated place for 3 to 4 days. About 9 to 12 small potatoes will yield 1 pound.

Exchanges: 3 Lean Meat, 2 Vegetable, 1-1/2 Fat, 1 Starch

Nutritional Information

Serving Size: 1/4 recipe
Calories: 391
Sodium: 183 mg
Cholesterol: 88 mg

Carbohydrate: 32 gm
Protein: 28 gm
Fat: 18 gm
Fiber: 5 gm

Garlic Rosemary Turkey

Cathy Dobbins, Rio Rancho, New Mexico

The house smells so good while this turkey is cooking that my family can hardly wait to eat! This is a beautiful, succulent main dish.

1 whole turkey (10 to 12 pounds)
6 to 8 garlic cloves
2 large lemons, halved
2 teaspoons dried rosemary, crushed
1 teaspoon rubbed sage
Low-Fat Gravy (recipe on page 305), optional

Cut six to eight small slits in turkey skin; insert garlic between the skin and meat. Squeeze two lemon halves inside the turkey and leave them inside. Squeeze remaining lemon over outside of turkey. Spray the turkey with nonstick cooking spray; sprinkle with rosemary and sage. Place on a rack in a roasting pan. Bake, uncovered, at 325° for 1 hour. Cover and bake 2-1/2 to 3-1/2 hours longer or until a meat thermometer reads 185°. Serve with gravy if desired. **Yield:** 12 servings.

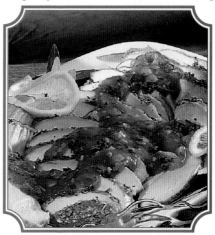

Exchanges: 4–1/2 Lean Meat

Nutritional Information

Serving Size: 1/12 recipe
Calories: 185
Sodium: 107 mg
Cholesterol: 98 mg

Carbohydrate: 1 gm
Protein: 33 gm
Fat: 4 gm
Fiber: trace
(Calculated without gravy)

Baked Lemon Chicken

Aida Babbel, Bowen Island, British Columbia

*I found this recipe many years ago when my children were toddlers.
I've changed it a little over the years to make it my own.
Everyone in my family just loves it!*

3 tablespoons all-purpose flour
1/4 teaspoon pepper
4 boneless skinless chicken
    breast halves (1 pound)
2 tablespoons vegetable oil
1 medium onion, chopped
1 tablespoon margarine
1 cup low-sodium chicken broth
3 tablespoons lemon juice
2 teaspoons dried basil
1/2 teaspoon dried thyme
4 lemon slices
2 tablespoons minced fresh
    parsley
2 cups hot cooked rice

In a shallow bowl, combine flour and pepper; set aside 1 tablespoon. Add chicken to the bowl and dredge in flour mixture. In a skillet, brown chicken in oil; transfer to an ungreased 9-in. square baking dish. In a saucepan, saute onion in margarine. Add reserved flour mixture; stir to form a thick paste. Gradually add broth, lemon juice, basil and thyme; mix well. Bring to a boil; cook and stir for 2 minutes or until thickened and bubbly. Pour over the chicken. Top each half with a lemon slice. Sprinkle with parsley. Cover and bake at 350° for 25-30 minutes or until the chicken juices run clear. Serve over rice. **Yield:** 4 servings.

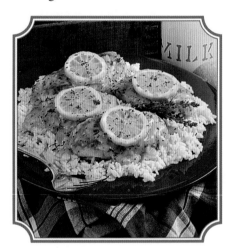

Exchanges: 3-1/2 Lean Meat, 1-1/2 Starch, 1/2 Vegetable

Nutritional Information

Serving Size: 1/4 recipe
Calories: 357
Sodium: 134 mg
Cholesterol: 67 mg

Carbohydrate: 31 gm
Protein: 30 gm
Fat: 11 gm
Fiber: 1 gm

Picante Chicken

Mary Henken, Alma, Illinois

I came up with this recipe after eating a similar dish in a Mexican restaurant. My family enjoys this one for its slightly spicy flavor...I like it's ease of preparation.

1 pound boneless skinless chicken breasts, cubed
1 tablespoon vegetable oil
1 cup chopped onion
1 cup chopped celery
1 cup chopped green *or* sweet red pepper
1 jar (12 ounces) picante sauce
1/2 teaspoon salt-free lemon-pepper seasoning
1/4 teaspoon salt-free seasoning blend
2 cups hot cooked rice

In a large skillet or wok, saute chicken in oil for 10-12 minutes or until juices run clear. Add onion, celery and pepper; saute until crisp-tender. Add picante sauce and seasonings; simmer for 30 minutes. Serve over rice. **Yield:** 4 servings.

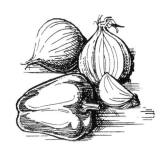

Exchanges: 3-1/2 Lean Meat, 1-1/2 Starch, 1 Vegetable, 1/2 Fat

Nutritional Information

Serving Size: 1/4 recipe
Calories: 327
Sodium: 764 mg
Cholesterol: 66 mg

Carbohydrate: 37 gm
Protein: 30 gm
Fat: 5 gm
Fiber: 2 gm

Turkey Burgers

Brenda Jones, Homestead, Florida

I created this recipe on a whim for company.
It was a hit. Now my family asks me quite often
to prepare these healthy, hearty burgers.

1 pound ground turkey breast
Egg substitute equal to 1 egg
1/4 cup dry bread crumbs
1 teaspoon steak sauce
1 teaspoon spicy brown
   mustard
1/4 teaspoon dried thyme
1/4 teaspoon pepper
4 hamburger buns, split
Lettuce leaves and tomato slices

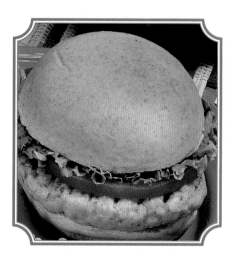

In a bowl, combine the first seven ingredients. Shape into four burgers (for easier shaping, use cold wet hands). Pan-fry, grill or broil until no longer pink. Serve on buns with lettuce and tomato. **Yield:** 4 servings.

Exchanges: 3-1/2 Lean Meat, 2-1/2 Starch

Nutritional Information

Serving Size: 1/4 recipe
Calories: 351
Sodium: 453 mg
Cholesterol: 71 mg

Carbohydrate: 36 gm
Protein: 37 gm
Fat: 6 gm
Fiber: 2 gm

Blackened Cajun Chicken

Marian Platt, Sequim, Washington

My son's a great cook who came up with this seasoning rub on his own. It's one of our favorite ways to prepare chicken because it's nice and zesty.

1 tablespoon *each* paprika, brown sugar, garlic powder and ground mustard
1 teaspoon *each* onion powder, ground cumin, dried thyme and pepper
1 teaspoon dried rosemary, crushed
1/2 to 1 teaspoon cayenne pepper
1 teaspoon salt-free seasoning blend
1 broiler/fryer chicken (3 pounds), cut up and skin removed

Combine all seasonings. Place chicken in a 13-in. x 9-in. x 2-in. baking dish; rub with half of the seasoning mixture. Cover and refrigerate overnight. Grill, covered, over medium heat, turning once, for 30-45 minutes or until juices run clear. **Yield:** 4 servings. **Editor's Note:** Seasoning mix is enough for two chickens. It may be made ahead and stored in an airtight container until needed.

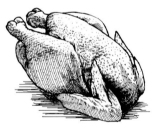

Exchanges: 3 Lean Meat, 2 Fat
Nutritional Information

Serving Size: 1/4 recipe
Calories: 276
Sodium: 81 mg
Cholesterol: 85 mg

Carbohydrate: 5 gm
Protein: 22 gm
Fat: 18 gm
Fiber: trace

Vegetable Chicken

Dorothy McGrew Hood, Northbrook, Illinois

The original recipe for this dish only called for vegetables, but I eventually added the chicken to make it a mouth-watering main meal.

1 broiler/fryer chicken (3 pounds), cut up and skin removed
2 cups sliced celery
2 cups fresh *or* frozen cut green beans
1-1/2 cups sliced carrots
1 large onion, sliced
1 small zucchini, diced
1 can (14-1/2 ounces) no-salt-added whole tomatoes, undrained and cut up
3 tablespoons quick-cooking tapioca
1 tablespoon sugar
1 teaspoon salt-free seasoning blend
1/2 teaspoon pepper

In an ungreased 13-in. x 9-in. x 2-in. baking dish, place chicken, celery, green beans, carrots and onion. In a small bowl, combine zucchini, tomatoes, tapioca, sugar, seasoning blend and pepper. Pour over chicken and vegetables. Cover tightly and bake at 350° for 1-1/2 hours or until chicken juices run clear and vegetable mixture thickens. Stir vegetables occasionally during baking. **Yield:** 4 servings.

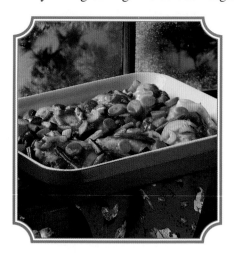

Exchanges: 3 Lean Meat, 3 Vegetable, 1-1/2 Fat, 1/2 Starch

Nutritional Information

Serving Size: 1/4 recipe
Calories: 376
Sodium: 162 mg
Cholesterol: 85 mg

Carbohydrate: 31 gm
Protein: 25 gm
Fat: 18 gm
Fiber: 6 gm

Garlic Chicken

Karen Kruckenberg, Harvard, Illinois

As a child, I spent countless hours with my mom in the kitchen.
Now I do the same with my own daughter.
Here's a dish I gradually developed through the years.

2 cups skim buttermilk
6 garlic cloves, minced
1 teaspoon Worcestershire
   sauce
1/2 teaspoon salt-free
   lemon-pepper seasoning
1/2 teaspoon pepper
1/4 teaspoon hot pepper sauce
1 broiler/fryer chicken (3 pounds),
   cut up and skin removed
Cayenne pepper

In a large resealable plastic bag or glass 13-in. x 9-in. x 2-in. baking dish, combine the first six ingredients. Add chicken pieces; turn to coat. Close bag or cover and refrigerate at least 8 hours. Drain and shake off excess marinade from chicken; do not rinse. Discard marinade. Sprinkle chicken lightly with cayenne pepper. Cover and grill over medium heat, turning once, for 30-45 minutes or until juices run clear. **Yield:** 4 servings.

BUYING GARLIC. Look for firm, plump bulbs with dry skins, avoiding those with soft or shriveled cloves. Unbroken bulbs can be stored in a cool, dry place for about 6 weeks. Once broken from the bulb, individual cloves should be used within a week.

Exchanges: 3 Lean Meat, 1-1/2 Fat, 1/2 Skim Milk

Nutritional Information

Serving Size: 1/4 recipe
Calories: 301
Sodium: 230 mg
Cholesterol: 89 mg

Carbohydrate: 8 gm
Protein: 25 gm
Fat: 18 gm
Fiber: trace

Grilled Chicken Kabobs

Sharon Hasty, New London, Missouri

We cook out all four seasons, so, I'm always in search of new marinades. We've been making these marvelous kabobs for years. They're a family favorite.

1/2 cup olive *or* vegetable oil
1/4 cup lemon juice
4 garlic cloves, minced
2 teaspoons honey
1-1/2 teaspoons dried thyme
1 teaspoon crushed red pepper flakes
1 teaspoon pepper
1 teaspoon salt-free seasoning blend
1 pound boneless skinless chicken breasts

In a small bowl, combine oil, lemon juice, garlic, honey, thyme, red pepper flakes, pepper and seasoning blend. Reserve half of marinade for basting; cover. Cut chicken into 1-in.-wide strips; weave on skewers. Place in an 11-in. x 7-in. x 2-in. glass baking dish. Pour remaining marinade over chicken. Cover and refrigerate for at least 4 hours. Drain, discarding marinade. Place skewers on grill over medium-low heat. Grill, turning and basting with reserved marinade, for 12 minutes or until juices run clear. **Yield:** 4 servings.

Exchanges: 3-1/2 Lean Meat, 1/2 Fat

Nutritional Information

Serving Size: 1/4 recipe
Calories: 201
Sodium: 76 mg
Cholesterol: 66 mg

Carbohydrate: 4 gm
Protein: 26 gm
Fat: 8 gm
Fiber: trace

Pork

*Satisfying pork and ham lend country-style
flair to these casseroles, skillet suppers,
hearty stews and grilled goodies.*

Herbed Pork Chops

Dianne Esposite, New Middletown, Ohio

Herbs are a fast and flavorful way to dress up pork.
Plus, they make the chops look so pretty on a platter.
I prepare these year-round as a way to capture the taste of summer.

4 boneless butterfly loin pork chops (4 ounces *each***)**
2 teaspoons lemon juice
2 tablespoons chopped fresh parsley
1/2 teaspoon dried rosemary, crushed
1/2 teaspoon dried thyme, crushed
1/4 teaspoon pepper

Brush pork chops with lemon juice. Combine seasonings; rub over chops. Grill, covered, over medium heat, turning occasionally, for 16-20 minutes or until juices run clear. **Yield:** 4 servings.

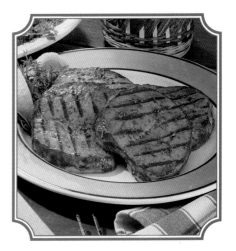

Exchanges: 3-1/2 Very Lean Meat, 1 Fat

Nutritional Information

Serving Size: 1/6 recipe
Calories: 161
Sodium: 53 mg
Cholesterol: 62 mg

Carbohydrate: trace
Protein: 25 gm
Fat: 6 gm
Fiber: trace

Ham and Red Beans

June Robinson, Bastrop, Louisiana

*I've cut some of the fat and calories from this traditional Southern dish.
But after one bite, you'll agree it still has plenty of flavor.*

**3 cans (16 ounces *each*) kidney
beans, rinsed and drained**
**1 can (14-1/2 ounces) Cajun *or*
Mexican stewed tomatoes**
**2 cups diced fully cooked
low-fat ham**
1/2 cup water
1/2 teaspoon garlic powder
1/2 teaspoon ground cumin
1/2 teaspoon dried thyme
1/2 teaspoon dried oregano
1/4 teaspoon pepper
3 dashes hot pepper sauce

In a large saucepan or Dutch oven, combine all ingredients; bring to a boil. Reduce heat; cover and simmer for 30 minutes. **Yield:** 10 servings.

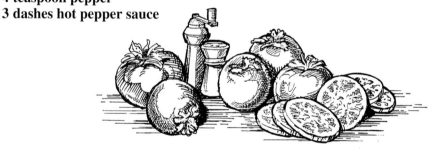

Exchanges: 2 Starch, 1-1/2 Lean Meat, 1/2 Vegetable

Nutritional Information

Serving Size: 3/4 cup
Calories: 235
Sodium: 514 mg
Cholesterol: 24 mg

Carbohydrate: 32 gm
Protein: 19 gm
Fat: 3 gm
Fiber: 12 gm

Low-Fat Fettuccine

Andrea Buchmann, Orlando, Florida

*This family favorite takes just minutes to prepare and
has a delightful combination of
noodles, ham, cheese and vegetables in a creamy sauce.*

12 ounces fettuccine
1 cup low-sodium chicken broth
2 garlic cloves, minced
1 cup quartered mushrooms
1/2 cup thinly sliced green onions
4 ounces fat-free cream
   cheese, cubed
4 ounces fully cooked low-sodium
   ham, cubed
1 cup quartered cherry tomatoes
1/2 cup grated Parmesan cheese
1/4 teaspoon white pepper

Cook the fettuccine according to package directions. In a saucepan over medium heat, bring broth and garlic to a boil. Add mushrooms and onions; reduce heat. Simmer, uncovered, for 3-5 minutes or until the mushrooms are tender. Add cream cheese and ham; cook and stir until cheese is melted. Add tomatoes; heat through. Remove from the heat; stir in Parmesan cheese and pepper. Rinse and drain fettuccine; top with the sauce. **Yield:** 5 servings.

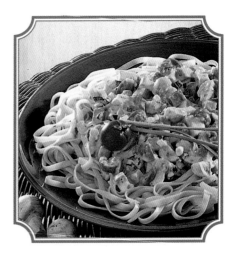

Exchanges: 2-1/2 Starch, 1-1/2 Lean Meat, 1/2 Vegetable

Nutritional Information

Serving Size: 1/5 recipe
Calories: 305
Sodium: 678 mg
Cholesterol: 22 mg

Carbohydrate: 43 gm
Protein: 20 gm
Fat: 7 gm
Fiber: 3 gm

Basil Baked Chops for Two

Dominique Petersen, Eden, Ontario

In this recipe, basil enhances the naturally delicious flavors of pork and vegetables. I like to make this dish during the summer months when fresh zucchini is abundant.

2 bone-in pork chops (5 ounces **each), trimmed**
1/4 teaspoon garlic powder
1/4 teaspoon pepper
2 cups sliced zucchini
1 cup thinly sliced carrots
2 tablespoons chopped onion
1 teaspoon dried basil

Place each pork chop in the center of an 18-in. x 12-in. piece of heavy-duty foil. Sprinkle with garlic powder and pepper. Top with zucchini, carrots and onion. Sprinkle with basil. Bring opposite long edges of foil together over the top of vegetables and fold down several times. Fold the short ends toward the food and crimp tightly to prevent leaks. Place foil pouches on a baking sheet. Bake at 350° for 45-55 minutes or until pork juices run clear and vegetables are tender. **Yield:** 2 servings.

TO PEEL OR NOT TO PEEL. The skin of summer squash such as zucchini, crookneck and pattypan is very thin and edible. So there's no need to peel it off before using the squash in recipes.

Exchanges: 3 Lean Meat, 1-1/2 Vegetable, 1 Fat

Nutritional Information

Serving Size: 1/2 recipe
Calories: 251
Sodium: 90 mg
Cholesterol: 78 mg

Carbohydrate: 12 gm
Protein: 33 gm
Fat: 8 gm
Fiber: 4 gm

Sweet 'n' Sour Pockets

Kathy Harris, Old Hickory, Tennessee

This recipe combines two great foods that are fabulous together—ham and pineapple. I first made these for a ladies luncheon and was asked many times for the recipe.

1/3 cup fat-free mayonnaise
1/3 cup nonfat sour cream
1/2 teaspoon Dijon mustard
 1 can (8 ounces) unsweetened
    pineapple tidbits, drained
 5 pita pocket breads (6 inches),
    halved
10 lettuce leaves
10 slices (1 ounce *each*) fully cooked
    low-sodium ham
1/2 cup chopped green pepper
1/2 cup chopped red onion

In a small bowl, combine mayonnaise, sour cream and mustard. Cover and refrigerate for 1 hour. Just before serving, stir pineapple into mayonnaise mixture. Fill each pita half with lettuce, ham, 2 tablespoons pincapple mixture, green pepper and onion. **Yield:** 5 servings.

LEFTOVER ONION? If a recipe only calls for a small amount of onion, tightly wrap the unused portion with the skin intact, refrigerate and use within 5 days.

Exchanges: 2-1/2 Starch, 1-1/2 Lean Meat, 1/2 Vegetable, 1/2 Fat

Nutritional Information

Serving Size: 1/5 recipe
Calories: 335
Sodium: 1,074 mg
Cholesterol: 31 mg

Carbohydrate: 52 gm
Protein: 20 gm
Fat: 4 gm
Fiber: 3 gm

Pork Chop Potato Bake

Ardis Henning, Montello, Wisconsin

*Folks who sample my cooking tease me and
say I should open a restaurant. But I'm happy just cooking
comforting meals like this for family and friends.*

6 bone-in pork chops (5 ounces
  each), trimmed
1 can (10-3/4 ounces) reduced-
  fat, reduced-sodium condensed
  cream of mushroom soup,
  undiluted
1 can (4 ounces) sliced mushrooms,
  drained
1/4 cup low-sodium chicken broth
1/2 teaspoon garlic powder
1/2 teaspoon Worcestershire sauce
1/4 teaspoon dried thyme
1 can (16 ounces) whole potatoes,
  drained
1 package (10 ounces) frozen peas,
  thawed
1 tablespoon diced pimientos

In a large nonstick skillet coated with nonstick cooking spray, brown chops on each
side. Place chops in an ungreased 13-in. x
9-in. x 2-in. baking pan. Combine the next
six ingredients; mix well. Pour over pork.
Cover and bake at 350° for 1 hour. Add
potatoes, peas and pimientos. Cover and
bake 15 minutes longer or until pork is
tender and vegetables are heated through.
Yield: 6 servings.

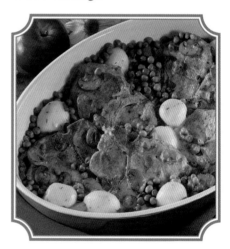

Exchanges: 4 Very Lean Meat, 1-1/2 Fat, 1 Starch, 1 Vegetable

Nutritional Information

Serving Size: 1/6 recipe
Calories: 307
Sodium: 732 mg
Cholesterol: 92 mg

Carbohydrate: 19 gm
Protein: 34 gm
Fat: 10 gm
Fiber: 4 gm

Pork and Pasta Stew

Margaret Bossuot, Carthage, New York

*You can make this stew in summer and use the
vegetables from your garden. Because it doesn't simmer for hours,
I often reach for this recipe when I need dinner in a hurry.*

1 pound lean boneless pork, cut
   into 1-inch strips
1/2 teaspoon salt-free lemon-pepper
   seasoning
1 tablespoon olive *or* vegetable oil
1 medium onion, sliced into thin
   wedges
1 garlic clove, minced
1 cup low-sodium chicken broth
3/4 cup salsa
1 tablespoon brown sugar
3 quarts water
1 teaspoon salt-free seasoning blend
1 package (8 ounces) spiral pasta
1 cup cut fresh green beans (1-inch
   pieces)
1 cup sliced yellow summer squash
1 cup sliced zucchini
1 cup sliced fresh mushrooms
1 tablespoon cornstarch
2 tablespoons cold water

Toss pork and lemon pepper; brown in oil in a nonstick skillet over medium heat. Add onion and garlic; saute until tender. Stir in broth, salsa and brown sugar; bring to a boil. Reduce heat; cover and simmer for 15-20 minutes or until pork is tender. Meanwhile, in a large saucepan over medium heat, bring water and seasoning blend to a boil. Add pasta and beans; return to a boil. Cook, uncovered, for 7 minutes. Add the squash, zucchini and mushrooms. Cook, uncovered, 6-7 minutes more or until pasta and vegetables are tender. Drain; set aside and keep warm. Combine cornstarch with cold water until smooth; add to the pork mixture and mix well. Bring to a boil; boil and stir for 2 minutes. To serve, place pasta and vegetables in a serving dish; top with pork mixture. **Yield:** 6 servings.

Exchanges: 2 Lean Meat, 2 Starch, 1-1/2 Vegetable, 1 Fat

Nutritional Information

Serving Size: 1/6 recipe
Calories: 321
Sodium: 213 mg
Cholesterol: 42 mg

Carbohydrate: 40 gm
Protein: 24 gm
Fat: 7 gm
Fiber: 4 gm

Pork Chops Deluxe

Sandy Krin, Watertown, Connecticut

With its one-pan convenience, I enjoy preparing this recipe often for hearty weekday meals.

6 boneless pork chops (4 ounces
  each), trimmed
2 tablespoons water
1 can (14-1/2 ounces) no-salt-added
  diced tomatoes
1 can (10-3/4 ounces) condensed
  golden mushroom soup,
  undiluted
1/3 cup chopped onion
2 teaspoons Dijon mustard
1 pound fresh mushrooms, sliced
1/4 teaspoon salt-free seasoning
  blend
3 cups hot cooked rice
2 tablespoons minced fresh parsley

In a nonstick skillet coated with nonstick cooking spray, brown pork chops on both sides. Remove and set aside. Add water, scraping bottom of the skillet to loosen any browned bits. Drain tomatoes, reserving juice; set tomatoes aside. Add juice, soup, onion, mustard, mushrooms and seasoning blend to skillet; mix well. Return chops to skillet. Cover and simmer for 30 minutes or until pork is tender. Stir in tomatoes; heat through. Combine rice and parsley. Serve the pork chops and sauce over rice. **Yield:** 6 servings.

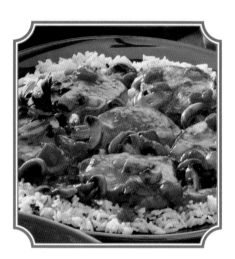

Exchanges: 3-1/2 Very Lean Meat, 2-1/2 Vegetable, 1 Starch, 1/2 Fat

Nutritional Information

Serving Size: 1/6 recipe
Calories: 320
Sodium: 493 mg
Cholesterol: 73 mg

Carbohydrate: 34 gm
Protein: 29 gm
Fat: 7 gm
Fiber: 2 gm

Apple-Topped Ham Steak

Eleanor Chore, Athena, Oregon

*Sweet apples combine nicely with tangy mustard in
this dish to create a luscious topping for skillet-fried ham steak.
It's great to serve this to guests in fall.*

1 fully cooked reduced-fat ham
   steak (2 pounds)
1 cup chopped onion
3 cups unsweetened apple juice
2 teaspoons Dijon mustard
2 medium green apples, cored and
   thinly sliced
2 medium red apples, cored and
   thinly sliced
2 tablespoons cornstarch
1/4 cup cold water
1 tablespoon minced fresh sage
  or 1 teaspoon rubbed sage
1/4 teaspoon pepper

In a large skillet coated with nonstick cooking spray, brown ham steak on both sides over medium heat; set aside and keep warm. In the same skillet, saute onion until tender. Stir in apple juice and mustard; bring to a boil. Add apples. Reduce heat; cover and simmer for 4 minutes or until apples are tender. Combine cornstarch and water until smooth; stir into apple juice mixture. Bring to a boil; boil and stir for 2 minutes. Stir in sage and pepper. Return ham steak to the skillet; heat through. **Yield:** 8 servings.

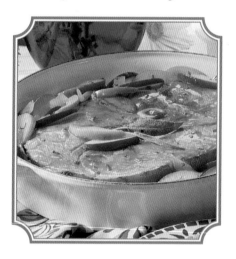

Exchanges: 2-1/2 Lean Meat, 1 Fruit, 1/2 Vegetable

Nutritional Information

Serving Size: 1/8 recipe
Calories: 236
Sodium: 1,478 mg
Cholesterol: 51 mg

Carbohydrate: 25 gm
Protein: 23 gm
Fat: 5 gm
Fiber: 2 gm

Garden Pork Skillet

Kathryn Bockus, Tuscumbia, Alabama

This is deliciously different than any other sweet-and-sour recipes because it's packed with produce. It makes a pretty presentation on the table, so it's great for special dinners.

1 pound lean boneless pork
1 can (8 ounces) unsweetened
  pineapple chunks
2 tablespoons light soy sauce
1-1/2 teaspoons ground ginger
1 garlic clove, minced
3 drops hot pepper sauce
1 cup julienned celery
1 cup julienned carrots
1 cup julienned green pepper
1 cup thinly sliced red onion
1/2 pound fresh mushrooms, sliced
1 cup julienned yellow squash
1 cup julienned zucchini
1 package (6 ounces) frozen
  snow peas

Cut pork into 1/8-in. x 1/2-in. x 2-in. strips; set aside. Drain juice from pineapple into a medium bowl; set pineapple aside. Add soy sauce, ginger, garlic and hot pepper sauce to juice; mix well. Add pork; cover and refrigerate at least 1 hour. With a slotted spoon, transfer pork to a large nonstick skillet coated with nonstick cooking spray. Brown pork over medium-high heat, stirring constantly; add marinade. Bring to a rolling boil for 1 minute. Reduce heat; cover and simmer for 20-25 minutes or until pork is tender. Add celery, carrots, green pepper and onion. Cook, uncovered, over medium heat until vegetables are crisp-tender. Add mushrooms, squash, zucchini, peas and pineapple; cook for 1-2 minutes or until vegetables are crisp-tender. **Yield:** 6 servings.

Exchanges: 2-1/2 Lean Meat, 2 Vegetable, 1/2 Fat

Nutritional Information

Serving Size: 1/6 recipe
Calories: 180
Sodium: 266 mg
Cholesterol: 42 mg

Carbohydrate: 16 gm
Protein: 20 gm
Fat: 5 gm
Fiber: 4 gm

Stuffed Ham Slices

Beverly Calfee, McDonald, Ohio

*Any occasion is perfect to present these tasty slices.
The great combination of a seasoned cheese spread,
hearty ham and zesty pickle appeals to folks of all ages.*

1 package (8 ounces) fat-free
cream cheese, softened
3/4 cup minced celery
1/2 cup shredded fat-free cheddar
cheese
1/3 cup minced fresh parsley
1/4 cup fat-free mayonnaise
2 tablespoons minced onion
1 unsliced loaf (1 pound)
Italian bread
8 slices (1 ounce *each*) fully
cooked low-sodium ham
4 whole low-sodium dill pickles,
sliced lengthwise

In a bowl, combine the first six ingredients. Cut bread in half lengthwise; spread each half with the cheese mixture. On the bottom half, layer half the ham, pickle slices and remaining ham. Replace top of loaf. Wrap tightly in plastic wrap; refrigerate for at least 2 hours before serving. **Yield:** 8 servings.

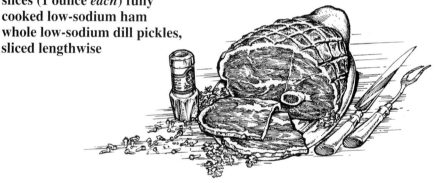

Exchanges: 2 Starch, 1-1/2 Lean Meat, 1/2 Vegetable

Nutritional Information

Serving Size: 1/8 recipe
Calories: 253
Sodium: 886 mg
Cholesterol: 18 mg

Carbohydrate: 35 gm
Protein: 18 gm
Fat: 4 gm
Fiber: 3 gm

Rosemary Pork Roast with Vegetables

Suzanne Strocsher, Bothell, Washington

*I found this recipe in a friend's collection years ago. Since then,
my family has requested it more times than I can count.*

2 garlic cloves, minced
5 teaspoons dried rosemary,
  crushed
4 teaspoons dried marjoram
1/2 teaspoon pepper
1 boneless pork loin roast (2-1/2
  pounds), trimmed
8 small red new potatoes,
  quartered
1 pound fresh baby carrots
1 tablespoon vegetable oil

In a small bowl, combine garlic, rosemary, marjoram and pepper; set aside 1 tablespoon. Rub remaining mixture over roast; place in a shallow roasting pan. Combine potatoes, carrots and oil in a large resealable plastic bag; add reserved spice mixture and toss to coat. Arrange vegetables around roast. Cover and bake at 325° for 1 hour. Uncover and bake 1 hour longer or until a meat thermometer reads 160°-170°. Let stand for 10 minutes before slicing. **Yield:** 8 servings.

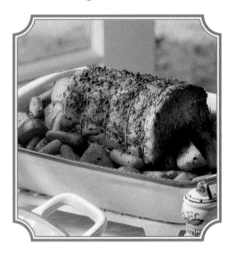

Exchanges: 3-1/2 Lean Meat, 1-1/2 Fat, 1/2 Vegetable

Nutritional Information

Serving Size: 1/8 recipe
Calories: 274
Sodium: 92 mg
Cholesterol: 78 mg

Carbohydrate: 14 gm
Protein: 32 gm
Fat: 9 gm
Fiber: 2 gm

Fruited Pork Picante

Anita Schebler, Phoenix, Arizona

*Colorful peaches, salsa, sweet red pepper and peas
make this dish attractive as well as great tasting. I received the
recipe from my mother-in-law, who's a great cook.*

1 pound boneless pork loin,
   trimmed and cut into
   1/2-inch cubes
1 tablespoon reduced-sodium taco
   seasoning mix
1 cup julienned sweet red pepper
1-1/2 cups salsa
   1/3 cup spreadable peach fruit
1 package (6 ounces) frozen
   snow peas

Toss pork with taco seasoning mix. In a nonstick skillet coated with nonstick cooking spray, brown pork over medium heat. Add red pepper; cook for 1 minute. Add salsa and preserves; mix well. Bring to a boil. Reduce heat; cover and simmer for 15-20 minutes or until pork is tender. Add peas; cook and stir over medium heat until tender. **Yield:** 4 servings.

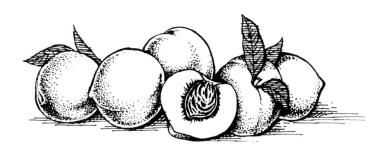

Exchanges: 4-1/2 Lean Meat, 1 Vegetable, 1 Fat, 1/2 Starch

Nutritional Information

Serving Size: 1 cup
Calories: 357
Sodium: 480 mg
Cholesterol: 90 mg

Carbohydrate: 12 gm
Protein: 35 gm
Fat: 11 gm
Fiber: 4 gm

Pork and Sweet Potatoes

Jean Christie, Penticton, British Columbia

*My family just loves sweet potatoes, so this is a perfect meal for us.
We like it best in fall, but it tastes terrific year-round.*

6 bone-in pork loin chops (5 ounces
  each)
1 tablespoon vegetable oil
1 cup orange juice
1 tablespoon brown sugar
1/4 teaspoon ground mace
1/4 to 1/2 teaspoon ground ginger
1/4 teaspoon salt-free seasoning blend
1/8 teaspoon pepper
2 large sweet potatoes (1-1/4 pounds)
2 tablespoons reduced-fat
  margarine, melted
2 teaspoons cornstarch
1 tablespoon water

In a skillet over medium heat, brown pork chops in oil. Place in a 13-in. x 9-in. x 2-in. baking pan coated with nonstick cooking spray. In a saucepan, combine orange juice, brown sugar, mace, ginger, seasoning blend and pepper; bring to a boil. Pour over chops. Cover and bake at 350° for 30 minutes. Peel potatoes; cut into 1/3-in. slices. Brush with margarine. Turn chops. Cover with potatoes; baste with pan juices. Cover and bake for 40 minutes longer or until potatoes are tender. Remove chops and potatoes to a serving platter; cover and keep warm. Combine cornstarch and water until smooth; stir into pan juices. Bring to a boil; cook and stir for 2 minutes or until thickened. Pour over pork chops and potatoes. **Yield:** 6 servings.

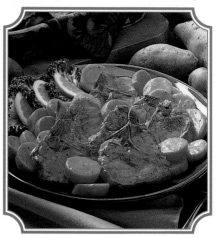

Exchanges: 4-1/2 Very Lean Meat, 1-1/2 Starch, 1-1/2 Fat

Nutritional Information

Serving Size: 1/6 recipe
Calories: 369
Sodium: 121 mg
Cholesterol: 78 mg

Carbohydrate: 30 gm
Protein: 33 gm
Fat: 13 gm
Fiber: 1 gm

Asparagus Lasagna

Jane Galvin, Englewood, Florida

Our family had an asparagus farm during the Depression.
This is one of the best ways Mother fixed it.

1 pound fresh asparagus, trimmed
2 garlic cloves, minced
1/2 teaspoon dried thyme
2 tablespoons margarine
2 tablespoons all-purpose flour
1-1/3 cups skim milk
Pepper to taste
    5 lasagna noodles, cooked and
    drained
    1 cup (4 ounces) shredded reduced-
    fat mozzarella cheese
    1 cup julienned fully cooked
    low-sodium ham

In a skillet, cook asparagus in a small amount of water until crisp-tender, about 6-8 minutes; drain and set aside. In a saucepan over medium heat, saute garlic and thyme in margarine. Stir in flour until blended. Gradually whisk in milk; bring to a boil. Cook and stir for 2 minutes or until thickened. Add pepper. Cut noodles in half; place four noodles in an 11-in. x 7-in. x 2-in. baking dish coated with nonstick cooking spray. Layer a third of the white sauce, mozzarella cheese, ham and asparagus over noodles. Top with three noodles and another layer of sauce, cheese, ham and asparagus. Repeat layers. Cover and bake at 350° for 30 minutes or until heated through. **Yield:** 4 servings.

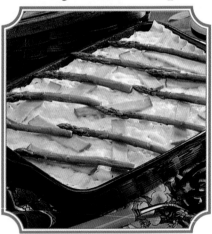

Exchanges: 2 Lean Meat, 2 Fat, 1–1/2 Vegetable, 1–1/2 Starch

Nutritional Information

Serving Size: 1/4 recipe
Calories: 367
Sodium: 783 mg
Cholesterol: 48 mg

Carbohydrate: 33 gm
Protein: 29 gm
Fat: 13 gm
Fiber: 2 gm

Hot Pot Stew

Sandra Allen, Leadville, Colorado

This full-bodied stew is ideal for chilly rainy days.
So I often try—unsuccessfully—to sneak some into the freezer
before my family can eat it all!

1 cup cubed lean boneless pork
(1/2-inch pieces)
1 cup cubed fully cooked low-
sodium ham
1 cup coarsely chopped green
pepper
1/2 cup chopped onion
1/2 cup chopped celery
1 garlic clove, minced
3 cups cubed red potatoes
3 cups water
1 can (16 ounces) pinto beans,
rinsed and drained
1 can (15.8 ounces) great northern
beans, rinsed and drained
1-1/4 teaspoons sugar
1 teaspoon low-sodium chicken
bouillon granules

1 teaspoon low-sodium beef
bouillon granules
1/4 teaspoon ground nutmeg
1/4 teaspoon coarsely ground pepper
1 package (10 ounces) frozen
chopped spinach

In a Dutch oven or soup kettle coated with nonstick cooking spray, brown pork over medium-high heat. Add ham, green pepper, onion, celery and garlic. Reduce heat to medium; cook for 8-10 minutes or until vegetables are just tender, stirring occasionally. Add the next nine ingredients. Reduce heat; cover and simmer for 20 minutes or until potatoes are tender. Add spinach and cook until heated through. **Yield:** 8 servings (2-1/2 quarts).

Exchanges: 2 Starch, 1-1/2 Lean Meat, 1 Vegetable

Nutritional Information

Serving Size: 1/8 recipe
Calories: 268
Sodium: 493 mg
Cholesterol: 31 mg

Carbohydrate: 38 gm
Protein: 22 gm
Fat: 4 gm
Fiber: 8 gm

Mexican Pork Stew

Mary Lou Kosanke, Hualapai, Arizona

I originally received this recipe from a friend.
To add a little zip, I stirred in some green chilies.
This Southwestern-style stew is super!

**2-1/2 pounds lean boneless pork, cut
into 1-inch cubes
1 garlic clove, minced
1 cup chopped onion
1 can (14-1/2 ounces) no-salt-
added whole tomatoes,
undrained and cut up
1 can (4 ounces) chopped green
chilies
1 tablespoon minced fresh
cilantro *or* parsley
2 teaspoons dried oregano
2 bay leaves
1 tablespoon cornstarch
1 tablespoon water**

In a large skillet coated with nonstick cooking spray, brown pork and garlic. Add onion; saute until tender. Stir in tomatoes, chilies, cilantro, oregano and bay leaves; cover and simmer for 40 minutes or until pork is tender and no longer pink. Combine cornstarch and water until smooth; add to skillet. Bring to a boil; boil for 2 minutes, stirring constantly. Discard bay leaves. **Yield:** 10 servings.

Exchanges: 3 Lean Meat, 1 Vegetable

Nutritional Information

Serving Size: 1/10 recipe
Calories: 168
Sodium: 196 mg
Cholesterol: 71 mg

Carbohydrate: 5 gm
Protein: 25 gm
Fat: 5 gm
Fiber: 1 gm

Cauliflower and Ham Casserole

Rosemary Flexman, Waukesha, Wisconsin

*My mother made this recipe many times when I was young.
I remember leaning on the table to watch her cook.*

1 tablespoon chopped onion
3 tablespoons margarine, *divided*
2 tablespoons all-purpose flour
1/2 teaspoon salt-free seasoning blend
Pepper to taste
1 cup skim milk
1/2 cup shredded reduced-fat
 cheddar cheese
1 medium head cauliflower, cut
 into florets, cooked and drained
2 cups cubed fully cooked
 low-sodium ham
1 jar (4-1/2 ounces) sliced
 mushrooms, drained
1 jar (2 ounces) diced pimientos,
 drained
6 saltines, crumbled

In a saucepan over medium heat, saute onion in 2 tablespoons of margarine until tender. Stir in flour, seasoning blend and pepper until smooth. Gradually add milk; cook and stir for 2 minutes or until thick and bubbly. Remove from the heat; stir in cheese until melted. Fold in cauliflower, ham, mushrooms and pimientos. Pour into a 2-qt. baking dish coated with nonstick cooking spray. In a small saucepan, brown cracker crumbs in remaining margarine; sprinkle over top. Cover and bake at 350° for 20 minutes. Uncover and bake 5-10 minutes longer or until heated through. **Yield:** 6 servings.

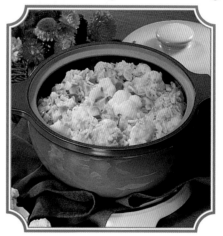

Exchanges: 2-1/2 Lean Meat, 2 Fat, 1 Vegetable

Nutritional Information

Serving Size: 1/6 recipe
Calories: 242
Sodium: 1,053 mg
Cholesterol: 43 mg

Carbohydrate: 14 gm
Protein: 23 gm
Fat: 10 gm
Fiber: 3 gm

Citrus Pork Roast

Irene Shiels, Wallingford, Connecticut

Wonderful herb and citrus flavors are light and delicious additions to a traditional pork roast. Guests will comment that this roast looks almost too good to eat.

1 medium grapefruit
1 medium orange
1 medium lemon
2 tablespoons olive *or* vegetable oil
1-1/2 teaspoons dried rosemary, crushed
1/2 teaspoon salt-free seasoning blend
1 garlic clove, minced
1 boneless pork loin roast (5 pounds), trimmed

Cut fruit in half; squeeze to remove juice, reserving rinds. In a large resealable plastic bag, combine fruit juices, oil, rosemary, seasoning blend and garlic. Make shallow cuts in top of roast. Place roast in bag; seal and turn to coat. Refrigerate overnight. Place roast and marinade in a shallow baking pan. Bake, uncovered, at 325° for 1-1/2 hours, basting with juices every 30 minutes. Meanwhile, slice fruit rinds into 1/4-in. strips; arrange around roast. Bake 30 minutes longer or until a meat thermometer reads 160°-170°. Let stand for 15 minutes before slicing. Arrange pork slices on a platter; drizzle with 1/4 cup of pan juices. **Yield:** 18 servings.

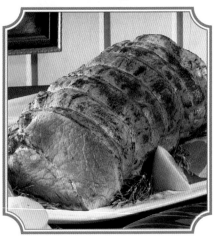

Exchanges: 3 Lean Meat, 1/2 Fat

Nutritional Information

Serving Size: 1/18 recipe
Calories: 186
Sodium: 65 mg
Cholesterol: 79 mg

Carbohydrate: 3 gm
Protein: 27 gm
Fat: 7 gm
Fiber: 1 gm

Oriental Pork with Hot Mustard Sauce

Alice Hoffman, Perry, Iowa

*You're not likely to have many leftovers when you
serve this taste-bud–tingling pork dish. Does it
ever go fast when I make it for a party!*

1 tablespoon ground mustard
1 teaspoon vegetable oil
1 teaspoon vinegar
1/8 teaspoon salt-free seasoning
blend
Dash ground turmeric
1/4 cup 2% milk
1/4 cup light soy sauce
2 tablespoons ketchup
1 tablespoon sugar
1/4 teaspoon molasses
1 garlic clove, crushed
2 pork tenderloins (1 pound *each*)
1 tablespoon sesame seeds,
toasted, optional

In a bowl, combine mustard, oil, vinegar, seasoning blend and turmeric; gradually add milk until smooth. Refrigerate. In a large resealable plastic bag or shallow glass dish, combine soy sauce, ketchup, sugar, molasses and garlic. Add pork; seal or cover and refrigerate for 4-6 hours, turning oc- casionally. Place the pork in a shallow roasting pan; discard marinade. Bake, un- covered, at 350° for 40 minutes or until a meat thermometer reads 160°-170°. Let stand for 5 minutes. Slice pork; sprinkle with sesame seeds if desired. Serve with the mustard sauce. **Yield:** 8 servings.

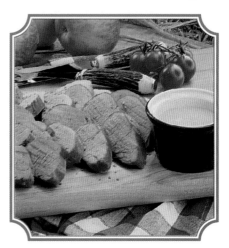

Exchanges: 3 Lean Meat, 1/2 Fat

Nutritional Information

Serving Size: 1/8 recipe
Calories: 184
Sodium: 409 mg
Cholesterol: 74 mg

Carbohydrate: 5 gm
Protein: 26 gm
Fat: 6 gm
Fiber: trace

Pork Chops Olé

Laura Turner, Channelview, Texas

This recipe is a fun and simple way to give pork chops south-of-the-border flair. The flavorful seasoning, rice and melted cheddar cheese make this dish a crowd-pleaser.

6 bone-in pork loin chops (5 ounces *each*)
1 tablespoon vegetable oil
1/8 teaspoon salt-free seasoning blend
1/8 teaspoon pepper
3/4 cup uncooked long grain rice
1-1/2 cups water
1 can (8 ounces) tomato sauce
1/2 envelope reduced-sodium taco seasoning mix (2 tablespoons)
1 medium green pepper, chopped
1/2 cup shredded reduced-fat cheddar cheese

In a large nonstick skillet, brown pork chops in oil; sprinkle with seasoning blend and pepper. Meanwhile, in a 13-in. x 9-in. x 2-in. baking dish coated with nonstick cooking spray, combine the rice, water, tomato sauce and taco seasoning; mix well. Arrange chops over rice; top with green pepper. Cover and bake at 350° for 1-1/2 hours. Uncover and sprinkle with cheese; return to the oven until cheese is melted. **Yield:** 6 servings.

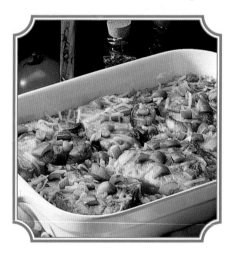

Exchanges: 2-1/2 Lean Meat, 1 Vegetable, 1 Starch, 1/2 Fat

Nutritional Information

Serving Size: 1/6 recipe
Calories: 273
Sodium: 324 mg
Cholesterol: 58 mg

Carbohydrate: 23 gm
Protein: 23 gm
Fat: 9 gm
Fiber: 1 gm

Garden Kabobs

Lorri Cleveland, Kingsville, Ohio

*When my garden is at its peak, I like to make this colorful entree.
Besides the great flavor, I also enjoy its easy preparation and cleanup.*

1/4 cup vegetable oil
1/4 cup lemon juice
1/4 cup light soy sauce
1/4 cup packed brown sugar
  2 garlic cloves, minced
  3 whole cloves
Dash dried basil
2-1/2 pounds pork tenderloin, cut
    into 1-1/4-inch pieces
  2 dozen cherry tomatoes
  2 dozen fresh mushroom caps
  1 large green *or* sweet red pepper,
    cut into 1-1/2-inch cubes
  2 small zucchini, cut into 1-inch
    slices
  1 medium onion, cut into wedges

In a bowl, combine first seven ingredients;
set aside. Assemble kabobs by threading
meat and vegetables on metal skewers.
Place in a large glass dish. Pour marinade
over kabobs; cover and refrigerate 6 hours
or overnight. Turn several times. To cook,
grill kabobs over hot heat until the meat
and vegetables have reached desired done-
ness. **Yield:** 10 servings.

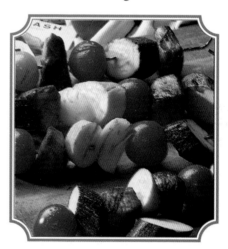

Exchanges: 3 Lean Meat, 1 Vegetable

Nutritional Information

Serving Size: 1/10 recipe
Calories: 189
Sodium: 125 mg
Cholesterol: 74 mg

Carbohydrate: 9 gm
Protein: 26 gm
Fat: 6 gm
Fiber: 2 gm

Pork with Mushroom Sauce

Dorothy Thompson, Chicago, Illinois

Treat your family to a festive meal of pork tenderloin without spending hours in the kitchen. It's easy enough to prepare for weekday dinners and impressive enough to serve on special occasions.

1 pork tenderloin (1 pound)
1/2 teaspoon dried thyme
1/2 teaspoon salt-free seasoning blend
1/4 teaspoon pepper
2 tablespoons reduced-fat margarine
1 cup sliced fresh mushrooms
1 small onion, sliced
1-1/2 teaspoons cornstarch
2/3 cup skim milk
1 tablespoon Dijon mustard

Cut tenderloin crosswise into fourths. Slice each piece in half but do not cut all the way through; open and flatten each piece. Combine the thyme, seasoning blend and pepper; sprinkle half over the pork. In a large nonstick skillet, cook pork in margarine for 3-4 minutes on each side. Add mushrooms and onion. Cook and stir until vegetables are almost tender and pork is no longer pink. Remove meat to a platter and keep warm. Combine the cornstarch, milk, mustard and remaining thyme mixture until smooth. Stir into vegetable mixture. Bring to a boil. Cook and stir for 2 minutes or until thickened. Spoon over pork and serve immediately. **Yield:** 4 servings.

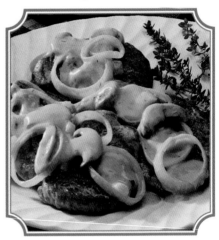

Exchanges: 3-1/2 Lean Meat, 1 Vegetable

Nutritional Information

Serving Size: 1/4 recipe
Calories: 209
Sodium: 240 mg
Cholesterol: 75 mg

Carbohydrate: 8 gm
Protein: 26 gm
Fat: 8 gm
Fiber: 1 gm

Sesame Pork Kabobs

Mildred Sherrer, Bay City, Texas

Our son and daughter-in-law discovered this recipe while living in Japan. Folks always comment on the wonderful marinade and crunchy sesame seeds.

3/4 cup finely chopped onion
1/2 cup light soy sauce
1/4 cup sesame seeds, toasted
1/4 cup water
3 tablespoons sugar
4-1/2 teaspoons minced garlic
1-1/2 teaspoons ground ginger
1/8 teaspoon cayenne pepper
2 pork tenderloins (3/4 pound *each*), trimmed

In a large resealable plastic bag or shallow glass container, combine the first eight ingredients. Cut pork across the grain into 1/4-in.-thick medallions; add to marinade and turn to coat. Seal bag or cover container; refrigerate for at least 1 hour. Drain and discard marinade. Accordion-fold each medallion, threading about 10 pieces each onto long skewers. Grill, uncovered, over medium coals, turning often, for 9-12 minutes or until meat is no longer pink. **Yield:** 6 servings.

GARLIC EQUATION. One medium garlic clove yields 1/2 teaspoon minced. You can also use minced garlic from a jar in any recipe calling for minced garlic.

Exchanges: 3 Lean Meat, 1 Fat, 1/2 Vegetable

Nutritional Information

Serving Size: 1/6 recipe
Calories: 216
Sodium: 261 mg
Cholesterol: 74 mg

Carbohydrate: 8 gm
Protein: 26 gm
Fat: 8 gm
Fiber: 2 gm

Oktoberfest Roast Pork

Carol Stevens, Basye, Virginia

We especially like this roast at our own Oktoberfest dinner.

1 pound dry navy beans
1 teaspoon rubbed sage
1 teaspoon salt-free seasoning
  blend
1/2 teaspoon pepper
1/8 teaspoon ground allspice
Dash cayenne pepper
1 boneless rolled pork loin roast
  (3 pounds)
2 tablespoons vegetable oil
2 tablespoons chopped fresh
  parsley
1/2 cup low-sodium chicken broth
2 medium tart apples, cut into
  wedges
1 large red onion, cut into wedges

Place beans in a Dutch oven or soup kettle; add water to cover by 2 in. Bring to a boil; boil for 2 minutes. Remove from the heat; cover and let stand for 1 hour. Meanwhile, combine sage, seasoning blend, pepper, allspice and cayenne; rub over roast. In a Dutch oven, brown roast in oil on all sides; drain. Drain beans and discard liquid; stir parsley into beans. Place beans around roast. Stir in broth. Cover and simmer for 2 hours or until a meat thermometer reads 150°. Place apples and onion on top of beans; cover and simmer for 30 minutes or until beans are tender and meat thermometer reads 160°-170°. Let stand 10-15 minutes before slicing. **Yield:** 12 servings.

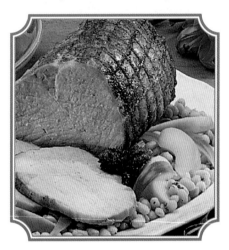

Exchanges: 3-1/2 Lean Meat, 1-1/2 Starch, 1 Fat, 1/2 Fruit

Nutritional Information

Serving Size: 1/12 recipe
Calories: 378
Sodium: 59 mg
Cholesterol: 67 mg

Carbohydrate: 27 gm
Protein: 32 gm
Fat: 16 gm
Fiber: 10 gm

Potluck Casserole

Janet Wielhouwer, Grand Rapids, Michigan

Whenever I take this dish to picnics and potlucks—which is quite often—people compare it to tuna noodle casserole. It reminds folks of Mom.

1/2 pound lean boneless pork, trimmed and cut into 3/4-inch cubes
1 cup sliced celery
1/4 cup chopped onion
2 tablespoons water
2 cups cooked no-yolk noodles
1 can (10-3/4 ounces) reduced-fat, reduced-sodium condensed cream of mushroom soup, undiluted
1 cup frozen peas
1/4 teaspoon salt-free seasoning blend
1/8 teaspoon pepper
3 tablespoons dry bread crumbs

In a skillet coated with nonstick cooking spray, brown the pork. Add celery, onion and water; cover and simmer for 1 hour or until pork is tender. Remove from the heat; add noodles, soup, peas, seasoning blend and pepper. Transfer to an ungreased 11-in. x 7-in. x 2-in. baking dish; sprinkle with crumbs. Bake, uncovered, at 350° for 20 minutes or until bubbly. **Yield:** 4 servings.

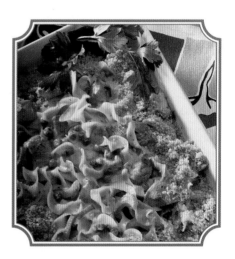

Exchanges: 2-1/2 Starch, 2 Lean Meat, 1 Vegetable, 1 Fat

Nutritional Information

Serving Size: 1/4 recipe
Calories: 381
Sodium: 679 mg
Cholesterol: 40 mg

Carbohydrate: 58 gm
Protein: 24 gm
Fat: 5 gm
Fiber: 6 gm

Zesty Pork Tenderloin

Sheryl Hurd-House, Fenton, Michigan

A zesty rub seasons pork tenderloin overnight for exceptional flavor. The next day, it bakes in no time. So it's easy to put a fast yet fancy meal on the table.

2 pork tenderloins (1 pound *each*), trimmed
1/3 cup olive *or* vegetable oil
1/4 cup minced fresh parsley
2 garlic cloves, minced
1 tablespoon grated fresh gingerroot *or* 1/2 teaspoon ground ginger
2 teaspoons dried oregano
2 teaspoons dried rosemary, crushed
1/2 teaspoon paprika
1/2 teaspoon salt-free seasoning blend
1/4 teaspoon pepper
1/4 teaspoon ground nutmeg

Place tenderloins in an ungreased 13-in. x 9-in. x 2-in. glass baking dish. Combine remaining ingredients; rub over tenderloins. Cover and refrigerate 6 hours or overnight. Bake, uncovered, at 425° for 25-30 minutes or until a meat thermometer reads 160°-170°. Let stand for 5 minutes before slicing. **Yield:** 8 servings.

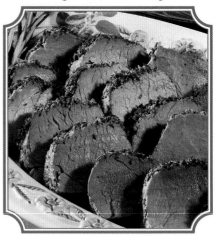

Exchanges: 3 Lean Meat, 1 Fat

Nutritional Information

Serving Size: 1/8 recipe
Calories: 217
Sodium: 58 mg
Cholesterol: 74 mg

Carbohydrate: trace
Protein: 24 gm
Fat: 13 gm
Fiber: trace

Citrus Pork Skillet

Shirley Nordblum, Youngsville, Pennsylvania

Our grandchildren often ask me to prepare this stir-fry when they come to visit, so I keep the recipe close at hand.

1/2 pound pork tenderloin, trimmed
1/2 to 3/4 teaspoon ground cumin
1/4 teaspoon pepper
1/4 teaspoon salt-free seasoning blend
2 garlic cloves, minced
1 cup low-sodium chicken broth
2/3 cup orange juice
2 tablespoons cider vinegar
1-1/2 teaspoons brown sugar
1 cup julienned carrots
2 tablespoons cornstarch
1/2 cup thinly sliced green onions

Cut pork into 1/2-in. x 1/2-in. x 2-in. strips. In a large resealable plastic bag, combine cumin, pepper and seasoning blend. Add pork; seal bag and shake to coat. In a large nonstick skillet coated with nonstick cooking spray, stir-fry pork and garlic over medium heat until pork is browned. In a bowl, combine broth, orange juice, vinegar and brown sugar; mix well. Add carrots and 1-1/2 cups of the broth mixture to skillet; bring to a boil. Reduce heat; cover and simmer for 5 minutes or until carrots are tender. Combine cornstarch and remaining broth mixture until smooth; add to skillet, stirring constantly. Bring to a boil; cook and stir for 2 minutes or until thickened. Add green onions; cook for 1 minute. **Yield:** 4 servings.

Exchanges: 1-1/2 Lean Meat, 1 Vegetable, 1/2 Fruit
Nutritional Information

Serving Size: 1/4 recipe
Calories: 138
Sodium: 71 mg
Cholesterol: 38 mg

Carbohydrate: 15 gm
Protein: 13 gm
Fat: 3 gm
Fiber: 2 gm

Mustard Pork Tenderloins

Diane Leskauskas, Chatham, New Jersey

Brushing these tasty pork medallions with mustard and coating them with seasoned dry bread crumbs before baking makes the meat tender and juicy.

1/2 cup dry bread crumbs
1/2 teaspoon dried thyme
1/4 teaspoon garlic powder
1/4 teaspoon onion powder
1-1/4 pounds pork tenderloin
1/4 cup Dijon mustard
1 tablespoon margarine, melted

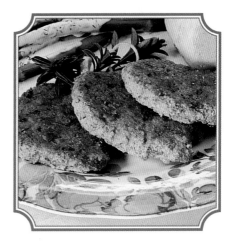

In a shallow bowl, combine the crumbs, thyme, garlic powder and onion powder; set aside. Cut tenderloin crosswise into 12 pieces; pound each piece to 1/4-in. thickness. Combine mustard and butter; brush on each side of pork, then coat with reserved crumb mixture. Place in a greased shallow baking pan. Bake, uncovered, at 425° for 10 minutes; turn and bake about 5 minutes more or until no longer pink. **Yield:** 4 servings.

Exchanges: 4 Lean Meat, 1 Fat
Nutritional Information

Serving Size: 1/4 recipe

Calories: 267

Sodium: 582 mg

Cholesterol: 92 mg

Carbohydrate: 12 gm

Protein: 33 gm

Fat: 9 gm

Fiber: 1 gm

Fish & Seafood

When from-the-sea fare makes an
appearance on your table, you're bound to
reel in rave reviews from all landlubbers!

Catfish Jambalaya

Mrs. Bill Saul, Macon, Mississippi

My family owns a catfish processing plant. This colorful,
zippy main dish is a great favorite of ours.

2 cups chopped onion
1/2 cup chopped celery
1/2 cup chopped green pepper
2 garlic cloves, minced
2 tablespoons margarine
1 can (10 ounces) diced tomatoes
   and green chilies, undrained
1 cup sliced fresh mushrooms
1/4 teaspoon cayenne pepper
1/2 teaspoon salt-free seasoning
   blend
1 pound catfish fillets, cubed
2 cups hot cooked rice

In a saucepan over medium-high heat, saute onion, celery, green pepper and garlic in margarine until tender, about 10 minutes. Add tomatoes, mushrooms, cayenne and seasoning blend; bring to a boil. Add catfish. Reduce heat; cover and simmer until fish flakes easily with a fork, about 10 minutes. Serve with rice. **Yield:** 4 servings.

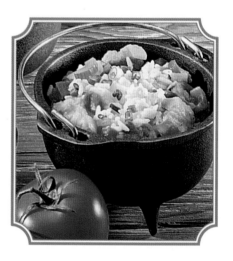

Exchanges: 3 Vegetable, 2-1/2 Lean Meat, 1 Fat, 1 Starch

Nutritional Information

Serving Size: 1/4 recipe
Calories: 356
Sodium: 428 mg
Cholesterol: 53 mg

Carbohydrate: 39 gm
Protein: 22 gm
Fat: 13 gm
Fiber: 3 gm

Baked Fish

Lynn Mathieu, Great Mills, Maryland

*I created this quick recipe after enjoying a seafood dish with
Parmesan cheese sprinkled on top at a restaurant.
The cheese added extra zip and gave me the idea to try it at home.*

**1/2 pound panfish fillets (perch, trout
 or whitefish)**
**4 teaspoons grated Parmesan
 cheese**
1/2 teaspoon dill weed

Place fish in a 10-in. pie plate coated with nonstick cooking spray. Sprinkle with Parmesan and dill. Bake, uncovered, at 350° for 8-10 minutes or until fish flakes easily with a fork. **Yield:** 2 servings.

FISH FACTS. When purchasing raw frozen fish, make sure it is solidly frozen. The wrapping should be free from tears and the fish shouldn't have an odor. Avoid fish with white, dark, icy or dry spots.

Exchanges: 3 Lean Meat
Nutritional Information

Serving Size: 1/2 recipe
Calories: 126
Sodium: 165 mg
Cholesterol: 51 mg

Carbohydrate: trace
Protein: 23 gm
Fat: 3 gm
Fiber: trace

Light Tuna Noodle Casserole

Sharen Oglesby, Anderson, California

*This recipe updates an old classic by using low-fat products.
It's a rich, creamy casserole that will satisfy the whole family.*

1 can (10-3/4 ounces) reduced-fat,
reduced-sodium condensed
cream of mushroom soup,
undiluted
2/3 cup water
1/2 cup skim milk
1/4 teaspoon ground mustard
1/8 teaspoon pepper
1/2 cup chopped celery
1/4 cup chopped green onions
  2 tablespoons olive *or*
  vegetable oil
  2 cans (6 ounces *each*) chunk light
  tuna in water, drained
1 container (8 ounces) egg
substitute
1 cup cooked no-yolk medium
noodles
1/2 cup shredded reduced-fat
cheddar cheese

In a large bowl, combine the soup, water, milk, mustard and pepper until blended. In a nonstick skillet, saute celery and onions in oil until celery is tender. Stir the vegetables, tuna, egg substitute and noodles into the soup mixture. Pour into a 2-qt. baking dish coated with nonstick cooking spray. Sprinkle with cheese. Bake at 375° for 50-60 minutes or until a knife inserted in the center comes out clean. **Yield:** 6 servings.

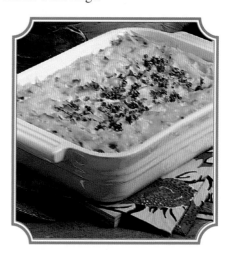

Exchanges: 3 Lean Meat, 1 Vegetable, 1 Starch

Nutritional Information

Serving Size: 1/6 recipe
Calories: 334
Sodium: 697 mg
Cholesterol: 22 mg

Carbohydrate: 34 gm
Protein: 28 gm
Fat: 8 gm
Fiber: 2 gm

Golden Baked Whitefish

Polly Habel, Monson, Massachusetts

This recipe represents our part of the country as fishing is very big here. We eat a lot of fish, and this is one of our favorite ways to prepare it.

2 pounds whitefish fillets
1/8 teaspoon pepper
1 egg white
1/2 teaspoon salt-free seasoning
   blend
1/4 cup reduced-fat mayonnaise
1/4 teaspoon dill weed
1 teaspoon dried minced onion
Fresh dill and lemon wedges,
   optional

Place fish in a 13-in. x 9-in. x 2-in. baking dish coated with nonstick cooking spray; sprinkle with pepper. Beat egg white with seasoning blend until stiff peaks form. Fold in mayonnaise, dill and onion; spoon over fish. Bake, uncovered, at 425° for 15-20 minutes or until topping is puffed and fish flakes easily with a fork. Garnish with dill and lemon if desired. **Yield:** 8 servings.

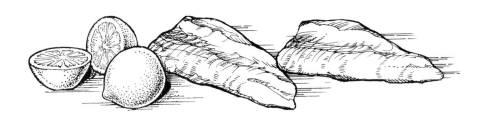

Exchanges: 3 Lean Meat

Nutritional Information

Serving Size: 1/8 recipe
Calories: 180
Sodium: 126 mg
Cholesterol: 68 mg

Carbohydrate: trace
Protein: 22 gm
Fat: 9 gm
Fiber: trace

Fish in Foil

Bill Davis, Casper, Wyoming

This recipe proves that cooking a satisfying supper can be fuss-free. Cooked this way, fish is moist and flavorful. Plus, there are no dishes to wash!

1 halibut steak (6 ounces)
4 medium mushrooms
2 cherry tomatoes, halved
2 lemon slices
1/2 medium green pepper, sliced
1/4 cup diet Mountain Dew
Crushed pepper

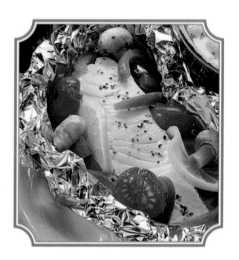

Place fish in the center of a 20-in. x 14-in. piece of heavy-duty foil. Place mushrooms, tomatoes, lemon and green pepper around fish. Fold edges of foil up; pour soda over fish. Fold foil to seal tightly. Bake at 375° for 20-25 minutes or until fish flakes easily with a fork. Open foil carefully to allow steam to escape. Sprinkle with pepper. **Yield:** 1 serving.

Exchanges: 5 Very Lean Meat, 2 Vegetable

Nutritional Information

Serving Size: 1 serving
Calories: 237
Sodium: 100 mg
Cholesterol: 54 mg

Carbohydrate: 11 gm
Protein: 38 gm
Fat: 5 gm
Fiber: 3 gm

Shrimp Salad Sandwiches

Saundra Woods, Woodbury, Tennessee

For years, my husband and sons were always ready to try new recipes. Now I have grandsons who love to come and eat at Grandma's house.

8 ounces cooked salad shrimp
3/4 cup chopped celery
2/3 cup fat-free mayonnaise
1 teaspoon dried minced onion
1/2 teaspoon dried tarragon, crushed
1/2 teaspoon hot pepper sauce
4 sandwich buns, split
Fresh spinach leaves

In a medium bowl, combine the first six ingredients; mix well. Refrigerate for at least 1 hour. Spoon 1/2 cup onto each bun; top with spinach leaves. **Yield:** 4 servings.

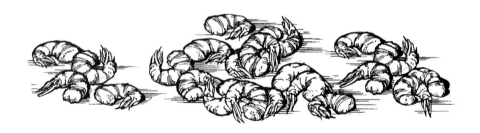

Exchanges: 2 Very Lean Meat, 1-1/2 Starch, 1/2 Fat
Nutritional Information
Serving Size: 1/4 recipe
Calories: 208
Sodium: 558 mg
Cholesterol: 104 mg

Carbohydrate: 23 gm
Protein: 18 gm
Fat: 4 gm
Fiber: trace

Baked Walleye

Joyce Szymanski, Monroe, Michigan

We live close to Lake Erie, which is nicknamed the "Walleye Capital of the World". I came up with this recipe as a way to serve that succulent fish.

3/4 cup chopped onion
3/4 cup chopped green pepper
3/4 cup chopped celery
 1 tablespoon dried parsley
   flakes
1/2 teaspoon garlic powder
1/2 teaspoon pepper
1/2 teaspoon salt-free seasoning
   blend
 1 cup low-sodium V-8 juice
 1 pound walleye fillets

In a saucepan, combine the first eight ingredients; bring to a boil. Reduce heat; simmer, uncovered, until vegetables are crisp-tender, stirring occasionally, about 5 minutes. Place fish in a 13-in. x 9-in. x 2-in. baking pan coated with nonstick cooking spray. Pour vegetable mixture over the fish. Cover and bake at 350° for 30 minutes or until fish flakes easily with a fork. **Yield:** 4 servings.

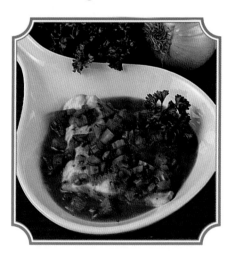

Exchanges: 3 Very Lean Meat, 1-1/2 Vegetable
Nutritional Information
Serving Size: 1/4 recipe
Calories: 144
Sodium: 216 mg
Cholesterol: 98 mg

Carbohydrate: 8 gm
Protein: 23 gm
Fat: 2 gm
Fiber: 1 gm

Oven-Fried Fish

Sandy Herman, Verona, Wisconsin

Parmesan cheese and special seasonings add a bit of an Italian flair to these fillets. Not only is this recipe low in fat, it's delicious as well. So it's sure to please everyone in the family.

1-1/2 pounds frozen cod *or* haddock fillets, thawed
2 tablespoons margarine, melted
1/2 cup seasoned bread crumbs
2 tablespoons grated Parmesan cheese
1 tablespoon dried parsley flakes
1/2 teaspoon Italian seasoning

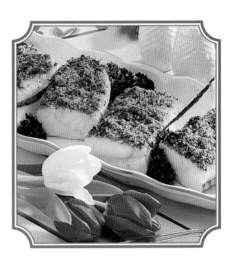

Cut fish into serving-size pieces; place in a 13-in. x 9-in. x 2-in. baking dish coated with nonstick cooking spray. Brush with margarine. Combine the remaining ingredients; sprinkle over fish. Bake, uncovered, at 425° for 10-15 minutes or until fish flakes easily with a fork. **Yield:** 4 servings.

Exchanges: 3 Very Lean Meat, 1 Fat, 1/2 Starch
Nutritional Information

Serving Size: 1/4 recipe
Calories: 208
Sodium: 573 mg
Cholesterol: 51 mg

Carbohydrate: 11 gm
Protein: 24 gm
Fat: 7 gm
Fiber: trace

Walleye Delight

Connie Reilly, Stanchfield, Minnesota

I love fish and think grilling is one of the best ways to prepare it. The combination of lemon juice, basil and other seasonings is fantastic.

1 pound walleye, pike, perch
   or trout fillets
2 teaspoons margarine,
   softened
1 tablespoon lemon juice
1 tablespoon snipped fresh basil
   or 1/2 to 1 teaspoon dried basil
1 teaspoon salt-free lemon-pepper
   seasoning
1/2 teaspoon garlic salt
4 ounces fresh mushrooms,
   sliced

Coat an 18-in. x 18-in. piece of heavy-duty foil with nonstick cooking spray. Place fillets on foil. Spread with margarine. Sprinkle with lemon juice, basil, lemon pepper and garlic salt. Top with mushrooms. Bring opposite edges of foil together; fold down several times. Fold remaining edges toward fish and seal tightly. Grill, covered, over hot heat for 10-14 minutes, turning once, or until fish flakes easily with a fork. **Yield:** 4 servings.

CARING FOR BASIL. Wrap fresh basil leaves in lightly damp paper towels, place in a plastic bag and refrigerate for up to 4 days. To store a bunch of fresh basil for up to a week, place stems in a glass of water. Cover the leaves with a plastic bag, securing the bag at the bottom with a rubber band.

Exchanges: 3 Very Lean Meat, 1/2 Vegetable

Nutritional Information

Serving Size: 1/4 recipe
Calories: 129
Sodium: 305 mg
Cholesterol: 97 mg

Carbohydrate: 2 gm
Protein: 22 gm
Fat: 3 gm
Fiber: trace

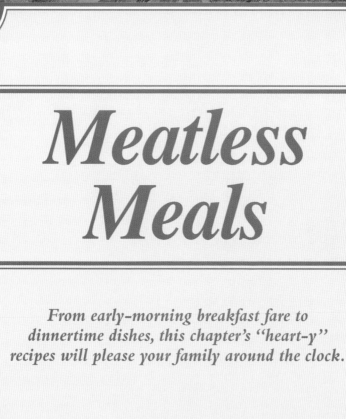

Meatless Meals

*From early-morning breakfast fare to
dinnertime dishes, this chapter's "heart-y"
recipes will please your family around the clock.*

Fresh Tomato Pasta Toss

Cheryl Travagliante, Independence, Ohio

I came up with this creation when my parent's tomato crop—and mine—were ready to harvest. My husband loves this dish.

3 pounds tomatoes
2 garlic cloves, minced
1 tablespoon vegetable oil
1 tablespoon minced fresh parsley
  or 1 teaspoon dried parsley
  flakes
1 tablespoon minced fresh basil
  or 1 teaspoon dried basil
2 teaspoons minced fresh
  oregano *or* 3/4 teaspoon
  dried oregano
1 teaspoon salt-free seasoning
  blend
1/8 teaspoon pepper
1/4 cup evaporated skim milk
1 pound tube pasta, cooked and
  drained
1/4 cup shredded Parmesan cheese

In a saucepan, bring water to a boil; dip tomatoes in water. Peel skins and discard. Chop pulp; set aside. In a skillet over medium heat, saute garlic in oil. Add tomato pulp, parsley, basil, oregano, seasoning blend and pepper; mix well. Bring to a boil; reduce heat. Add milk; heat through. Pour over hot pasta and toss to coat. Sprinkle with cheese. **Yield:** 8 servings.

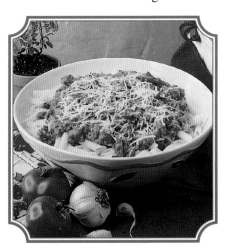

Exchanges: 2-1/2 Starch, 1-1/2 Vegetable, 1/2 Fat

Nutritional Information

Serving Size: 1/8 recipe
Calories: 282
Sodium: 82 mg
Cholesterol: 3 mg

Carbohydrate: 47 gm
Protein: 14 gm
Fat: 4 gm
Fiber: 3 gm

Multigrain Pancakes

Ann Harris, Lancaster, California

My husband and I love foods prepared with whole grains. But our children prefer white bread. So I created this recipe to appeal to their love of pancakes while giving them a taste of whole grain cooking.

1/2 cup all-purpose flour
1/4 cup whole wheat flour
1/4 cup cornmeal
 2 tablespoons sugar
1/2 teaspoon baking soda
1/2 teaspoon salt
 1 egg
 1 cup buttermilk
 2 tablespoons margarine, melted

In a large bowl, combine dry ingredients. In a small bowl, beat egg; add buttermilk and margarine. Stir into dry ingredients just until moistened. Pour batter by 1/4 cupfuls onto a hot nonstick griddle coated with nonstick cooking spray; turn when bubbles form on top of pancakes. Cook until second side is golden brown. **Yield:** 4 servings.

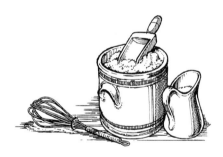

Exchanges: 2 Starch, 1 Fat

Nutritional Information

Serving Size: 2 pancakes
Calories: 227
Sodium: 586 mg
Cholesterol: 55 mg

Carbohydrate: 33 gm
Protein: 7 gm
Fat: 7 gm
Fiber: 2 gm

Tomato-Zucchini Pasta Supper

Donna Kohls, New Berlin, Wisconsin

The hearty taste of fresh ingredients makes this delicious as any you'll find in a fancy restaurant. I'm sure your family will love it as much as mine does!

1 medium onion, chopped
2 garlic cloves, minced
2 tablespoons olive *or* vegetable oil
2 cups cubed peeled fresh tomatoes
4 small zucchini, julienned
2 tablespoons chopped fresh basil
1/2 teaspoon salt-free seasoning blend
1/4 teaspoon pepper
12 ounces linguini *or* spaghetti, cooked and drained

In a large nonstick skillet, saute onion and garlic in oil until tender. Add tomatoes and zucchini; saute until tender. Add basil, seasoning blend and pepper. Serve over hot pasta. **Yield:** 4 servings.

OLIVE OIL TERMS. Extra-virgin describes the highest-quality (and most expensive) olive oil. Next, in order of descending quality, are superfine, fine and virgin. Pure olive oil is the least flavorful and least expensive.

Exchanges: 2 Vegetable, 1-1/2 Starch, 1 Fat
Nutritional Information

Serving Size: 1/4 recipe
Calories: 219
Sodium: 11 mg
Cholesterol: 0 mg
Carbohydrate: 33 gm
Protein: 6 gm
Fat: 8 gm
Fiber: 3 gm

Corn-Stuffed Peppers

Suzanne Hubbard, Greeley, Colorado

These peppers can be served alone as a meal or alongside pork chops, steak and hamburgers. I haven't had any complaints since creating this recipe years ago.

4 medium green peppers
1 can (10-3/4 ounces) reduced-fat, reduced-sodium condensed cream of celery soup, undiluted
2-1/2 cups frozen loose-pack hash brown potatoes, thawed
2 cups frozen corn, thawed
1/2 cup shredded reduced-fat cheddar cheese
1/4 cup chopped onion
1 jar (2 ounces) diced pimientos, drained
2 tablespoons snipped fresh chives
1/2 teaspoon salt-free seasoning blend

Slice tops off peppers and reserve; remove seeds. In a bowl, combine the remaining ingredients. Spoon filling into peppers and replace tops. Place in an 8-in. square baking dish; cover with foil. Bake at 350° for 45-60 minutes. **Yield:** 4 servings.

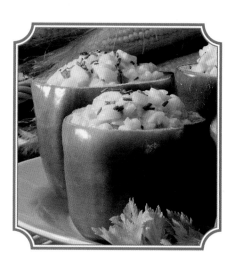

Exchanges: 2 Vegetable, 1-1/2 Starch, 1/2 Lean Meat, 1/2 Fat

Nutritional Information

Serving Size: 1/4 recipe
Calories: 219
Sodium: 610 mg
Cholesterol: 6 mg

Carbohydrate: 41 gm
Protein: 9 gm
Fat: 4 gm
Fiber: 5 gm

Freezer French Toast

Diane Perry, Castro Valley, California

*I keep a freezer full of these slices and simply pop them into
the oven for a homemade breakfast in no time.
My family prefers them over frozen store-bought French toast.*

Egg substitute equivalent to 4 eggs
  1 cup skim milk
Sugar substitute equivalent to 1
  tablespoon sugar
  1 teaspoon vanilla extract
  1/4 teaspoon ground nutmeg
  10 slices day-old low-fat French
  bread (3/4 inch thick)
  1 tablespoon margarine, melted

In a large bowl, beat egg substitute, milk, sugar substitute, vanilla and nutmeg. Place bread in a 13-in. x 9-in. x 2-in. baking dish coated with nonstick cooking spray. Pour egg mixture over bread. Let soak for several minutes, turning bread once to coat. Freeze until firm. Package in airtight containers. To bake, place bread on a well-greased baking sheet. Dot with margarine. Bake at 450° for 7 minutes; turn and bake 10-12 minutes longer or until golden brown. **Yield:** 5 servings.

MAKE-AHEAD MEAL. When you have extra time on your hands—and extra room in your freezer—consider doubling this recipe for Freezer French Toast. That way, you'll have enough slices for several breakfasts.

Exchanges: 2 Starch, 1 Lean Meat

Nutritional Information

Serving Size: 2 slices
Calories: 217
Sodium: 437 mg
Cholesterol: 1 mg

Carbohydrate: 30 gm
Protein: 12 gm
Fat: 5 gm
Fiber: 2 gm

Zucchini Pasta Casserole

Nettie Gornick, Butler, Pennsylvania

My husband is the gardener in our family, and I love to create new recipes with produce. I developed this dish during an especially bountiful zucchini harvest.

1 cup diced zucchini
1/2 cup diced green pepper
1/2 cup diced sweet red pepper
1/4 cup diced onion
1 tablespoon vegetable oil
1/4 cup dry bread crumbs
1/4 teaspoon salt-free seasoning blend
1/8 teaspoon pepper
1 cup cooked tricolor spiral pasta
2 tablespoons nonfat Parmesan cheese topping

In a small nonstick skillet, saute vegetables in oil until tender, about 7 minutes. Stir in the bread crumbs, seasoning blend and pepper; cook for 2-3 minutes. Remove from the heat; stir in pasta. Pour into a 1-qt. baking dish coated with non-stick cooking spray. Sprinkle with cheese topping. Bake, uncovered, at 375° for 10 minutes or until heated through. **Yield:** 2 servings.

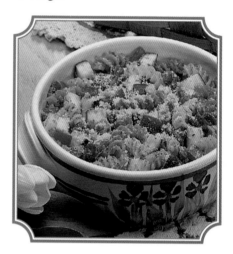

Exchanges: 2 Starch, 1 Vegetable, 1 Fat, 1/2 Lean Meat

Nutritional Information

Serving Size: 1/2 recipe
Calories: 277
Sodium: 238 mg
Cholesterol: 5 mg

Carbohydrate: 38 gm
Protein: 9 gm
Fat: 10 gm
Fiber: 4 gm

Egg and Tomato Scramble

Ilva Jasica, St. Joseph, Michigan

My mother used to make this for me as a special breakfast when I was a little girl. I think of her every time I prepare it these days.

1 plum tomato, peeled and chopped
1 teaspoon chopped fresh basil *or* 1/4 teaspoon dried basil
1 egg
1 teaspoon water
1 garlic clove, minced
1/8 teaspoon salt-free seasoning blend
Pepper to taste
1 slice bread, toasted

In a small bowl, combine tomato and basil; set aside. In another bowl, beat the egg, water, garlic, seasoning blend and pepper. In a small nonstick skillet coated with nonstick cooking spray, cook and stir egg mixture over medium heat until egg is nearly set. Add the tomato mixture; cook and stir until eggs are set. Serve with toast. **Yield:** 1 serving.

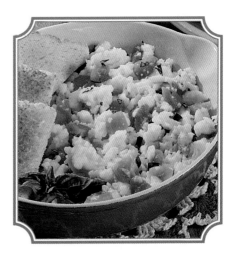

Exchanges: 1 Starch, 1 Meat, 1/2 Fat

Nutritional Information

Serving Size: 1 recipe
Calories: 197
Sodium: 69 mg
Cholesterol: 212 mg

Carbohydrate: 25 gm
Protein: 10 gm
Fat: 6 gm
Fiber: 1 gm

Garden Casserole

Phyllis Hickey, Bedford, New Hampshire

This casserole includes a medley of eggplant, zucchini and tomatoes.

2 pounds eggplant, peeled
2 tablespoons olive *or* vegetable oil
2 medium onions, finely chopped
2 garlic cloves, minced
2 medium zucchini, sliced 1/2 inch thick
5 medium tomatoes, peeled and chopped
2 celery ribs, sliced
1/4 cup minced fresh parsley
1/4 cup minced fresh basil *or* 1 tablespoon dried basil
1 teaspoon salt-free seasoning blend
1/2 teaspoon pepper
1/2 cup grated Romano cheese
1 cup dry bread crumbs
2 tablespoons margarine, melted
1 cup (4 ounces) shredded reduced-fat mozzarella cheese

Cut eggplant into 1/2-in.-thick slices, then cut into 1/2-in. cubes. In a nonstick skillet, saute eggplant in oil until lightly browned, about 5 minutes. Add onions, garlic and zucchini; cook 3 minutes. Add tomatoes, celery, parsley, basil, seasoning blend and pepper; bring to a boil. Reduce heat; cover and simmer for 10 minutes. Remove from the heat; stir in Romano cheese. Pour into a 13-in. x 9-in. x 2-in. baking dish coated with nonstick cooking spray. Combine crumbs and margarine; sprinkle on top. Bake, uncovered, at 375° for 15 minutes. Sprinkle with mozzarella cheese. Return to the oven for 5 minutes or until cheese is melted. **Yield:** 12 servings.

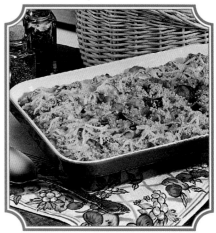

Exchanges: 2 Vegetable, 1 Fat, 1/2 Starch

Nutritional Information

Serving Size: 1/12 recipe
Calories: 134
Sodium: 161 mg
Cholesterol: 4 mg

Carbohydrate: 17 gm
Protein: 5 gm
Fat: 6 gm
Fiber: 4 gm

Basil Spaghetti Sauce

Marlane Jones, Allentown, Pennsylvania

My homemade sauce is packed with fresh tomatoes and assorted seasonings. Folks who sample it never seem to miss the meat.

1 cup chopped onion
8 garlic cloves, minced
1/4 cup vegetable oil
8 cups coarsely chopped peeled fresh tomatoes (about 5 pounds)
1/3 cup minced fresh basil *or* 2 tablespoons dried basil
1/4 cup minced fresh parsley
1-1/2 teaspoons salt-free seasoning blend
1/2 teaspoon pepper
1/2 teaspoon sugar
1 package (16 ounces) spaghetti, cooked and drained

In a large saucepan or Dutch oven over medium heat, saute onion and garlic in oil until tender. Add tomatoes, basil, parsley, seasoning blend, pepper and sugar; bring to a boil. Reduce heat; cover and simmer for 1-1/2 hours. Serve over spaghetti. **Yield:** 8 servings.

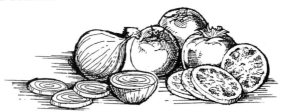

Exchanges: 2-1/2 Starch, 2 Vegetable, 1-1/2 Fat

Nutritional Information

Serving Size: 1/8 recipe
Calories: 314
Sodium: 20 mg
Cholesterol: 0 mg

Carbohydrate: 52 gm
Protein: 9 gm
Fat: 8 gm
Fiber: 5 gm

Zucchini Pizza

Joyce Sitz, Wichita, Kansas

Everyone enjoys the flavor of this delicious and different way to serve zucchini. It is a healthy, quick meal to prepare and a change from what we know as pizza. Guests will never guess what the "secret ingredient" is!

3 cups shredded zucchini
Egg substitute equivalent to 3 eggs
1/3 cup all-purpose flour
1-1/2 teaspoons dried oregano, *divided*
1 teaspoon dried basil, *divided*
1/4 teaspoon salt-free seasoning blend
2/3 cup sliced green onions
1/2 cup sliced ripe olives
1/2 cup chopped green pepper
2 cups (8 ounces) shredded reduced-fat mozzarella cheese
3 medium fresh tomatoes, peeled and thinly sliced

Press excess liquid from zucchini and place in a bowl. Add egg substitute, flour, 1/2 teaspoon oregano, 1/2 teaspoon basil and seasoning blend; mix well. Spread evenly over the bottom of a 13-in. x 9-in. x 2-in. baking dish coated with nonstick cooking spray. Bake at 450° for 8-10 minutes. Remove from oven and cool on a wire rack. Reduce heat to 350°. Sprinkle zucchini crust with green onions, olives, green pepper, cheese and remaining oregano and basil. Cover with tomato slices. Bake for 25-30 minutes or until cheese is bubbly. Cool on wire rack 5 minutes before cutting. **Yield:** 6 servings.

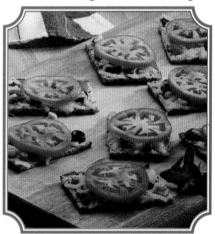

Exchanges: 2 Lean Meat, 1 Vegetable, 1/2 Starch, 1/2 Fat

Nutritional Information

Serving Size: 1/6 recipe
Calories: 198
Sodium: 359 mg
Cholesterol: 21 mg

Carbohydrate: 14 gm
Protein: 16 gm
Fat: 9 gm
Fiber: 3 gm

Asparagus Breakfast Strata

Maryellen Hays, Fort Wayne, Indiana

Filled with tasty ingredients like mushrooms, cheddar cheese and asparagus, this dish makes for hearty fare. You can prepare it the night before for a no-fuss breakfast, brunch or dish to pass.

Egg substitute equivalent to 8 eggs
 3 cups skim milk
 1 tablespoon Dijon mustard
 2 teaspoons dried basil
 2 tablespoons margarine, melted
 2 tablespoons all-purpose flour
 2 cups (8 ounces) shredded reduced-fat cheddar cheese
 1 package (10 ounces) frozen cut asparagus, thawed *or* 2 cups cut fresh asparagus, cooked
 2 cups sliced fresh mushrooms
 10 cups cubed reduced-calorie bread

In a large bowl, beat egg substitute, milk, mustard and basil. Gently stir in remaining ingredients until well mixed. Pour into a 13-in. x 9-in. x 2-in. baking dish coated with nonstick cooking spray. Cover and refrigerate 8 hours or overnight. Remove from the refrigerator 30 minutes before baking. Bake, uncovered, at 350° for 1 hour or until a knife inserted near the center comes out clean. Let stand 5 minutes before cutting. **Yield:** 12 servings.

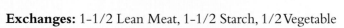

Exchanges: 1-1/2 Lean Meat, 1-1/2 Starch, 1/2 Vegetable

Nutritional Information

Serving Size: 1/12 recipe
Calories: 228
Sodium: 450 mg
Cholesterol: 6 mg

Carbohydrate: 26 gm
Protein: 17 gm
Fat: 6 gm
Fiber: 2 gm

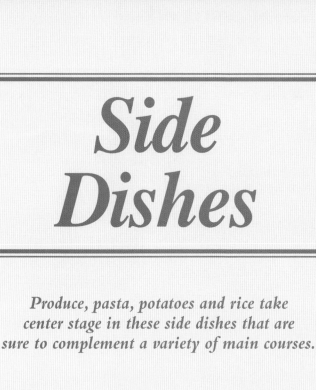

Side Dishes

Produce, pasta, potatoes and rice take center stage in these side dishes that are sure to complement a variety of main courses.

Festive Green Beans

Frances Janssen, Canyon Lake, Texas

For a vegetable dish that sports pretty colors, this one can't be beat. This dish has zip and gets people coming back for seconds.

1 pound fresh *or* frozen cut green beans
1/2 cup water
1/2 teaspoon salt-free seasoning blend
1/4 teaspoon pepper
1/2 teaspoon garlic powder
3/4 cup Mexican stewed tomatoes

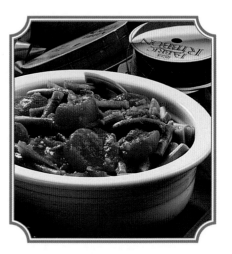

Cut beans into 2-in. pieces; place in a saucepan. Add water and seasoning blend; bring to a boil. Reduce heat and simmer 15 minutes or until tender; drain. Add the pepper, garlic powder and tomatoes; heat through. **Yield:** 6 servings.

Exchanges: 1-1/2 Vegetable

Nutritional Information

Serving Size: 1/2 cup
Calories: 34
Sodium: 62 mg
Cholesterol: 0 mg

Carbohydrate: 8 gm
Protein: 2 gm
Fat: trace
Fiber: 1 gm

Spiced Baked Beets

Margery Richmond, Lacombe, Alberta

Especially during fall and winter, this recipe is a favorite. With its red color, it looks great served at Christmastime. It's nice for taking to potlucks as well.

**4 cups shredded peeled beets
(about 4 to 5 medium)**
1 medium onion, shredded
1 medium potato, shredded
3 tablespoons brown sugar
3 tablespoons vegetable oil
2 tablespoons water
1 tablespoon vinegar
1/2 teaspoon salt-free seasoning blend
1/4 teaspoon pepper
1/4 teaspoon celery seed
1/8 to 1/4 teaspoon ground cloves

In a large bowl, combine beets, onion and potato; set aside. In a small bowl, combine brown sugar, oil, water, vinegar and seasonings. Pour over vegetables; toss to coat. Pour into a 1-1/2-qt. baking dish coated with nonstick cooking spray. Cover and bake at 350° for 45 minutes, stirring occasionally. Uncover and bake 15-25 minutes longer or until vegetables are tender. **Yield:** 10 servings.

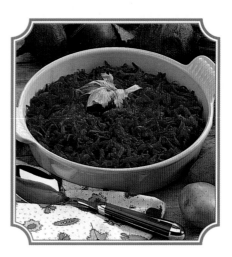

Exchanges: 1 Vegetable, 1 Fat

Nutritional Information

Serving Size: 1/10 recipe
Calories: 82
Sodium: 28 mg
Cholesterol: 0 mg

Carbohydrate: 11 gm
Protein: 1 gm
Fat: 4 gm
Fiber: 2 gm

Broccoli Noodle Side Dish

Louise Saluti, Sandwich, Massachusetts

*Colorful and satisfying, this dish can be
pulled together in a matter of minutes.
It makes a nice addition to any meaty meal.*

**6 cups (8 ounces) uncooked
no-yolk wide noodles**
3 to 4 garlic cloves, minced
**2 tablespoons olive *or*
vegetable oil**
**4 cups broccoli florets (about 1
pound)**
**1/2 pound fresh mushrooms,
thinly sliced**
1/2 teaspoon dried thyme
1/4 teaspoon pepper
**1 teaspoon salt-free seasoning
blend**

Cook noodles according to package directions. Meanwhile, in a nonstick skillet, saute garlic in oil until tender. Add broccoli; saute for 4 minutes or until crisp-tender. Add mushrooms, thyme, pepper and seasoning blend; saute for 2-3 minutes.

Drain noodles; add to broccoli mixture. Stir gently over low heat until heated through. **Yield:** 8 servings.

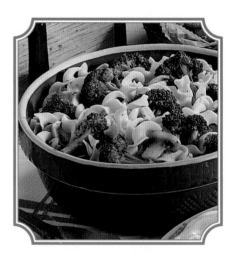

Exchanges: 1 Vegetable, 1 Fat, 1/2 Starch

Nutritional Information

Serving Size: 1/8 recipe
Calories: 160
Sodium: 39 mg
Cholesterol: 0 mg

Carbohydrate: 25 gm
Protein: 6 gm
Fat: 4 gm
Fiber: 3 gm

Chunky Applesauce

Judy Robertson, Southington, Connecticut

This sweet applesauce almost tastes like apple pie without the crust! My family can't resist digging into this side dish at dinnertime.

30 medium tart apples, peeled and quartered (about 11 pounds)
4 cups water
2 tablespoons ground cinnamon
Sugar substitute equivalent to 8 teaspoons sugar

Place apples and water in a large kettle. Cover and cook over medium-low heat for 30-40 minutes or until apples are tender; remove from the heat. Using a potato masher, mash apples to desired consistency. Stir in cinnamon and sugar substitute. Serve warm or cold. **Yield:** 14 cups.

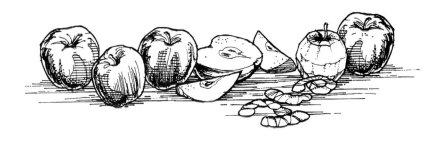

Exchanges: 1 Fruit

Nutritional Information

Serving Size: 1/2 cup
Calories: 66
Sodium: 1 mg
Cholesterol: 0 mg

Carbohydrate: 19 gm
Protein: trace
Fat: trace
Fiber: 3 gm

Chive Carrots

Dorothy Pritchett, Wills Point, Texas

With such rich garden-fresh flavor, you'll never guess how inexpensive this dish is to prepare. My husband and I both love the garlic in these colorful carrots.

1 pound carrots, cut into 2-inch julienne strips
1 garlic clove, minced
1 tablespoon vegetable oil
1 tablespoon margarine
2 tablespoons minced fresh chives *or* parsley

In a large nonstick skillet, saute carrots and garlic in oil and margarine for 3 minutes. Reduce heat; cover and cook for 10 minutes or until carrots are crisp-tender. Sprinkle with chives. Serve immediately. **Yield:** 4 servings.

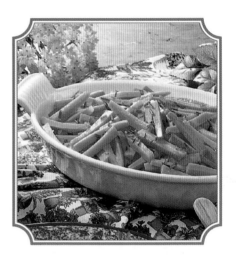

Exchanges: 2-1/2 Vegetable, 1 Fat

Nutritional Information

Serving Size: 1/4 recipe
Calories: 103
Sodium: 68 mg
Cholesterol: 0 mg

Carbohydrate: 12 gm
Protein: 1 gm
Fat: 6 gm
Fiber: 3 gm

Fancy Brussels Sprouts

Dorothy Anderson, Ottawa, Kansas

This is a simple and tasty way to dress up brussels sprouts. The parsley, sugar and crisp water chestnuts make the sprouts fresh tasting and festive looking.

1 cup water
1/4 cup minced fresh parsley
Sugar substitute equivalent to 1
  teaspoon sugar
1/2 teaspoon salt-free seasoning
  blend
2 pints fresh brussels sprouts,
  halved *or* 2 packages (10
  ounces *each*) frozen brussels
  sprouts, thawed
1 can (8 ounces) water
  chestnuts, drained and diced
1 tablespoon margarine

In a saucepan over medium heat, bring water, parsley, sugar substitute and seasoning blend to a boil. Add brussels sprouts. Cover and simmer for 6-8 minutes or until tender; drain. Add water chestnuts and margarine; heat through. **Yield:** 6 servings.

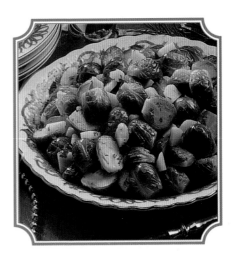

Exchanges: 2-1/2 Vegetable

Nutritional Information

Serving Size: 1/6 recipe
Calories: 74
Sodium: 34 mg
Cholesterol: 0 mg

Carbohydrate: 12 gm
Protein: 4 gm
Fat: 2 gm
Fiber: 6 gm

Baked Vidalia Onion

Norma Durham, Rogersville, Tennessee

*Served alongside a variety of fish and meat, this
tender onion is a nice change of pace. Folks
find it a fun and flavorful side dish.*

1 medium Vidalia *or* sweet onion
2 teaspoons margarine
1/4 teaspoon salt-free seasoning
blend
Pepper to taste

Quarter onion halfway through and open slightly. Place on an 18-in. x 12-in. piece of heavy-duty foil. Place margarine in center of onion; sprinkle with seasonings. Fold foil to seal tightly. Bake at 350° for 60-70 minutes or until onion is tender. Open foil carefully to allow steam to escape. **Yield:** 1 serving.

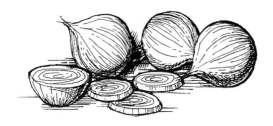

Exchanges: 4 Vegetable, 1/2 Fat

Nutritional Information

Serving Size: 1 recipe
Calories: 132
Sodium: 93 mg
Cholesterol: 0 mg

Carbohydrate: 21 gm
Protein: 3 gm
Fat: 5 gm
Fiber: 3 gm

Dilled Corn and Peas

Marlene Muckenhirn, Delano, Minnesota

Celebrate the harvest season with this striking combination of crisp colorful vegetables. Seasoned with dill, margarine and seasonings, it's an easy but impressive addition to any meal.

2-1/2 cups fresh *or* frozen sugar snap peas
2 cups fresh *or* frozen corn
1 small sweet red pepper, julienned
1/4 cup water
1 tablespoon margarine
1 teaspoon minced fresh dill *or* 1/4 teaspoon dill weed
1/8 teaspoon salt-free seasoning blend
1/8 teaspoon pepper

Place peas, corn, red pepper and water in a saucepan; cover and cook over high heat for 2-4 minutes or until vegetables are crisp-tender. Drain. Add margarine, dill, seasoning blend and pepper; toss to coat. **Yield:** 8 servings.

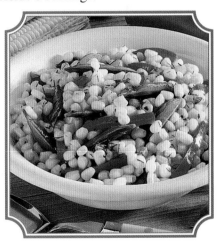

Exchanges: 1 Starch

Nutritional Information

Serving Size: 1/2 cup
Calories: 75
Sodium: 60 mg
Cholesterol: 0 mg

Carbohydrate: 14 gm
Protein: 3 gm
Fat: 2 gm
Fiber: 3 gm

Oven-Roasted Potato Wedges

Ellen Benninger, Stoneboro, Pennsylvania

Rosemary lends a delicious, delicate flavor to these potato wedges. This recipe is elegant enough for company, yet easy enough for every day.

4 unpeeled baking potatoes
 (2 pounds)
2 tablespoons olive *or* vegetable oil
1 medium onion, chopped
2 garlic cloves, minced
1 tablespoon minced fresh
 rosemary *or* 1 teaspoon dried
 rosemary, crushed
1/2 teaspoon salt-free seasoning
 blend
1/4 teaspoon pepper

Cut potatoes lengthwise into wedges; place in a 13-in. x 9-in. x 2-in. baking pan coated with nonstick cooking spray. Drizzle with oil. Sprinkle with onion, garlic, rosemary, seasoning blend and pepper; stir to coat. Bake, uncovered, at 400° for 45-50 minutes or until tender, turning once. **Yield:** 8 servings.

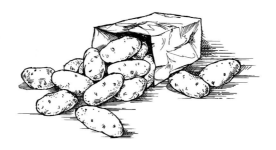

Exchanges: 1 Starch, 1 Fat

Nutritional Information

Serving Size: 1/8 recipe
Calories: 115
Sodium: trace
Cholesterol: 0 mg

Carbohydrate: 22 gm
Protein: 3 gm
Fat: 3 gm
Fiber: 3 gm

Hot Vegetable Plate

Julie Polakowski, West Allis, Wisconsin

A creamy mustard sauce adds spark to an interesting lineup of vegetables in this fall side dish. You'll always receive compliments with this special presentation.

1 medium kohlrabi
1 medium turnip
1 small rutabaga
4 medium carrots, halved crosswise
4 medium leeks (white portion only), sliced
12 fresh cauliflowerets
MUSTARD SAUCE:
  1/4 cup margarine
  2 tablespoons all-purpose flour
Pinch pepper
  1 cup skim milk
  1 to 2 teaspoons Dijon mustard

Peel kohlrabi, turnip and rutabaga; cut into 1/4-in. slices. Halve the kohlrabi and turnip slices; quarter the rutabaga slices. Place all vegetables in a large saucepan and cover with water; cook until crisp-tender. Meanwhile, melt margarine in a small saucepan; stir in flour until smooth. Add pepper. Gradually add milk; cook and stir until mixture boils. Reduce heat; cook and stir for 1 minute or until thickened. Remove from the heat; stir in mustard. Drain vegetables; serve with warm mustard sauce. **Yield:** 8 servings.

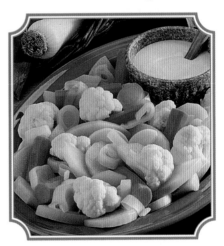

Exchanges: 2 Vegetable, 1 Fat, 1/2 Starch

Nutritional Information

Serving Size: 1/8 recipe with 2 tablespoons sauce
Calories: 135
Sodium: 137 mg
Cholesterol: trace

Carbohydrate: 22 gm
Protein: 4 gm
Fat: 4 gm
Fiber: 4 gm

Vegetable Kabobs with Rice

Nancy Johnson, Connersville, Indiana

My husband and I like gardening, and these kabobs are a fun way to enjoy our fresh vegetables. They're so easy to make and they can grill right along with the main course.

1/2 cup fat-free Italian salad dressing
1 tablespoon minced fresh parsley
1 teaspoon dried basil
2 medium yellow squash, cut into 1-inch pieces
8 small boiling onions, peeled
8 cherry tomatoes
8 medium fresh mushrooms
2 cups hot cooked rice (without added salt)

In a small bowl, combine dressing, parsley and basil. Alternate the vegetables on eight skewers. Place on a grill rack over medium-hot heat. Baste with dressing mixture and turn frequently for 15 minutes or until vegetables are tender. To serve, place 1/2 cup rice on each plate and top with two kabobs. **Yield:** 4 servings.

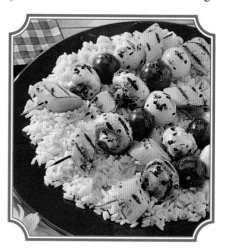

Exchanges: 2 Vegetable, 1-1/2 Starch
Nutritional Information

Serving Size: 1/4 recipe
Calories: 190
Sodium: 301 mg
Cholesterol: 0 mg

Carbohydrate: 41 gm
Protein: 6 gm
Fat: trace
Fiber: 5 gm

Chilly Dilly Carrots

Lizzie Sartin, Brookhaven, Mississippi

I serve these carrots often, since they're so nutritious and versatile. This dish is my favorite. It can be made a few days ahead of time, so it's easy when you're planning to serve it for a special meal.

1/2 pound carrots, sliced
2 tablespoons fat-free Italian salad dressing
2 tablespoons fat-free ranch salad dressing
2 tablespoons chopped onion
1-1/2 teaspoons minced fresh dill *or* 1/2 teaspoon dill weed
1-1/2 teaspoons minced fresh parsley *or* 1/2 teaspoon dried parsley flakes
1 teaspoon sugar
1/8 teaspoon salt-free seasoning blend
Dash pepper

Place carrots in a small saucepan and cover with water; cook until crisp-tender. Drain and place in a small bowl. Combine remaining ingredients; pour over carrots.

Cover and refrigerate for 6 hours or overnight, stirring occasionally. **Yield:** 2 servings.

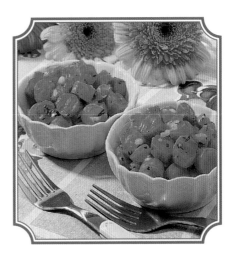

Exchanges: 2-1/2 Vegetable

Nutritional Information

Serving Size: 1/2 recipe
Calories: 87
Sodium: 340 mg
Cholesterol: 0 mg

Carbohydrate: 20 gm
Protein: 1 gm
Fat: trace
Fiber: 4 gm

Barley and Corn Casserole

Diane Molberg, Emerald Park, Saskatchewan

This hearty, colorful casserole goes well with chicken, pork or fish. For convenience, it can easily be made ahead and refrigerated before serving.

3 garlic cloves, minced
1 cup chopped onion
2/3 cup chopped carrots
1 tablespoon vegetable oil
3 cups low-sodium chicken broth
1 cup regular pearl barley
1/4 teaspoon salt-free seasoning
    blend
1/8 teaspoon pepper
2 cups frozen corn, thawed
1/2 cup chopped fresh parsley

In a nonstick skillet over medium heat, saute the garlic, onion and carrots in oil until tender. Transfer to a 2-qt. baking dish coated with nonstick cooking spray; add broth, barley, seasoning blend and pepper. Mix well. Cover and bake at 350° for 1 hour. Stir in corn and parsley. Cover and bake 10-15 minutes more or until the barley is tender and corn is heated through. **Yield:** 12 servings.

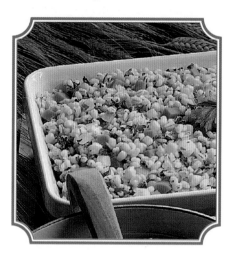

Exchanges: 1 Vegetable, 1 Starch

Nutritional Information

Serving Size: 1/2 cup	Carbohydrate: 22 gm
Calories: 113	Protein: 4 gm
Sodium: 34 mg	Fat: 2 gm
Cholesterol: 1 mg	Fiber: 4 gm

Herbed Wild Rice

David Collin, Martinez, California

Like many cooking enthusiasts, I've discovered good food pleases the palate and soothes the soul! This rice has a nice nutty flavor and the wonderful aroma of sage.

1 cup sliced green onions
2 tablespoons margarine
1 cup uncooked wild rice
3 cups low-sodium chicken broth
1 teaspoon rubbed sage
3/4 teaspoon dried thyme
1/2 teaspoon salt-free seasoning blend

In a saucepan over medium heat, saute the onions in margarine until tender, about 5 minutes. Add rice; cook for 8-10 minutes. Add broth, sage, thyme and seasoning blend. Pour into an ungreased 1-1/2-qt. baking dish. Cover and bake at 350° for 70-80 minutes or until rice is tender and liquid is absorbed. **Yield:** 8 servings.

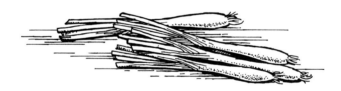

Exchanges: 1 Starch, 1/2 Fat

Nutritional Information

Serving Size: 1/8 recipe
Calories: 109
Sodium: 71 mg
Cholesterol: 1 mg

Carbohydrate: 16 gm
Protein: 4 gm
Fat: 3 gm
Fiber: 2 gm

Root Vegetable Medley

Marilyn Smudzinski, Peru, Illinois

*Equally good with turkey, pork or beef, this dish is
one my husband requests at least once a month.*

6 small red potatoes, quartered
**1 medium rutabaga, peeled and
cut into 1-inch cubes**
**3 medium carrots, cut into 1/2-inch
slices**
**1 medium turnip, peeled and cut
into 1-inch cubes**
**1 to 2 medium parsnips, peeled and
cut into 1/2-inch slices**
1 medium onion, cut into eighths
GLAZE:
    1 tablespoon margarine
    3 tablespoons brown sugar
    1 teaspoon cornstarch
1/4 cup water
    3 tablespoons lemon juice
1/2 teaspoon dill weed
1/2 teaspoon salt-free seasoning blend
1/8 teaspoon pepper

Place potatoes and rutabaga in a large
saucepan; cover with water. Bring to a
boil. Reduce heat; cover and simmer for
8 minutes. Add remaining vegetables; re-turn to a boil. Reduce heat; cover and simmer for 10 minutes or until vegetables are
tender; drain. For glaze, melt margarine in
a saucepan; stir in brown sugar and cornstarch until smooth. Stir in water, lemon
juice, dill, seasoning blend and pepper;
bring to a boil. Cook and stir for 2 minutes.
Pour over vegetables and toss to coat.
Yield: 8 servings.

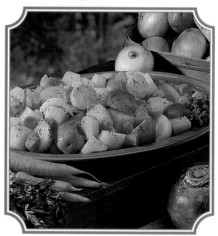

Exchanges: 2 Vegetable, 1 Starch, 1/2 Fat

Nutritional Information

Serving Size: 1 cup
Calories: 144
Sodium: 61 mg
Cholesterol: 0 mg

Carbohydrate: 32 gm
Protein: 4 gm
Fat: 1 gm
Fiber: 5 gm

Minty Peas and Onions

Santa D'Addario, Brooklyn, New York

My mother always relied on peas and onions when she was in a hurry and needed a quick side dish. Besides being easy to prepare, this dish was loved by everyone in our family.

2 large onions, cut into 1/2-inch wedges
1/2 cup chopped sweet red pepper
2 tablespoons vegetable oil
2 packages (16 ounces *each*) frozen peas
2 tablespoons minced fresh mint *or* 2 teaspoons dried mint

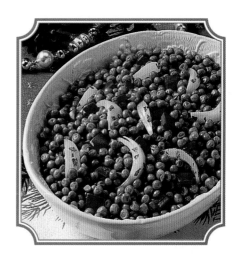

In a large nonstick skillet, saute onions and red pepper in oil until onions just begin to soften. Add peas; cook, uncovered, stirring occasionally, for 10 minutes or until heated through. Stir in mint and cook for 1 minute. **Yield:** 8 servings.

Exchanges: 1 Vegetable, 1 Starch, 1 Fat

Nutritional Information

Serving Size: 1/8 recipe
Calories: 143
Sodium: 129 mg
Cholesterol: 0 mg

Carbohydrate: 22 gm
Protein: 7 gm
Fat: 4 gm
Fiber: 6 gm

Microwave Spaghetti Squash

Lina Vainauskas, Shaw Air Force Base, South Carolina

One of the pleasant surprises about squash is that it's so low in calories.
That means I can "splurge" a little with the other ingredients.
Spaghetti squash is fun to work with and so tender and tasty!

**1 spaghetti squash (about
  1-1/2 pounds)
1 medium sweet red pepper,
  thinly sliced
1 small onion, thinly sliced
2 garlic cloves, minced
1 tablespoon olive *or* vegetable oil
1 medium tomato, chopped
1 medium zucchini, thinly sliced
1 cup sliced fresh mushrooms
1 tablespoon cider *or* tarragon
  vinegar
1 teaspoon dried tarragon
1/2 teaspoon salt-free seasoning
  blend
1/4 teaspoon pepper**

Pierce squash with a fork. Place on paper towel in microwave; cook on high for 6 minutes per pound or until squash is soft. Let stand for 5-10 minutes. Cut in half; remove seeds and scoop out pulp. Set aside. In a 2-qt. microwave-safe casserole, toss red pepper, onion, garlic and olive oil. Cover and microwave on high for 2 minutes or until slightly soft. Add tomato, zucchini, mushrooms, vinegar, tarragon, seasoning blend and pepper. Cover and microwave on high for 3 minutes or until crisp-tender. Toss with squash and serve immediately. **Yield:** 6 servings. **Editor's Note:** This recipe was tested in a 700-watt microwave.

Exchanges: 2 Vegetable, 1/2 Fat

Nutritional Information

Serving Size: 1/6 recipe	Carbohydrate: 14 gm
Calories: 80	Protein: 2 gm
Sodium: 23 mg	Fat: 3 gm
Cholesterol: 0 mg	Fiber: 3 gm

Potato Pockets

Denise Nebel, Wayland, Iowa

Our sons like to help me assemble potatoes, carrots and onions into foil packages that we can put on the grill. The sprinkling of cheese adds a nice touch.

4 medium potatoes, julienned
3 carrots, julienned
1/3 cup chopped red onion
2 tablespoons margarine
1/2 teaspoon salt-free seasoning blend
1/8 teaspoon pepper
1/4 cup shredded Parmesan cheese

Divide the potatoes, carrots and onion equally between four pieces of heavy-duty aluminum foil (about 18 in. x 12 in.). Top with margarine; sprinkle with seasoning blend and pepper. Bring opposite short ends of foil together over vegetables and fold down several times. Fold unsealed ends toward vegetables and crimp tightly. Grill, covered, over medium heat for 20 minutes or until potatoes are tender. Re-move from grill. Open foil and sprinkle with cheese; reseal for 5 minutes or until the cheese melts. **Yield:** 4 servings.

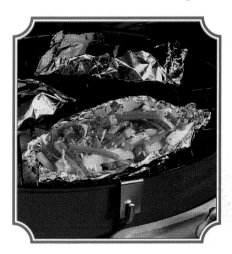

Exchanges: 1-1/2 Starch, 1 Vegetable, 1 Fat

Nutritional Information

Serving Size: 1/4 recipe
Calories: 205
Sodium: 202 mg
Cholesterol: 5 mg

Carbohydrate: 33 gm
Protein: 8 gm
Fat: 7 gm
Fiber: 5 gm

Mushroom Potatoes

Skip Dolliver, South Hamilton, Massachusetts

*I frequently serve these as a change from mashed potatoes.
Our son thinks this creamy casserole is absolutely delicious.*

1 can (10-3/4 ounces) reduced-fat,
  reduced-sodium condensed
  cream of mushroom soup,
  undiluted
1/2 cup skim milk
1 large onion, chopped
4 medium potatoes, peeled, diced
  and cooked
Paprika

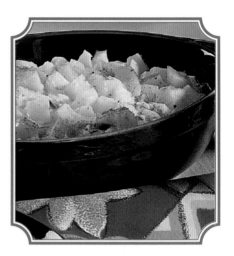

In a bowl, combine soup, milk and onion.
Stir in the potatoes. Pour into a 1-1/2-qt.
baking dish coated with nonstick cooking
spray. Sprinkle with paprika. Bake, uncovered, at 350° for 30 minutes or until
bubbly. **Yield:** 8 servings.

Exchanges: 1 Vegetable, 1 Starch

Nutritional Information

Serving Size: 1/8 recipe

Calories: 89

Sodium: 264 mg

Cholesterol: 2 mg

Carbohydrate: 19 gm

Protein: 3 gm

Fat: 1 gm

Fiber: 2 gm

Spanish Rice

Jerri Moror, Rio Rancho, New Mexico

The carrots, peas and tomatoes make this rice so pretty.
This versatile side dish goes especially well with a Mexican meal,
but you can successfully serve it with any entree.

1 cup uncooked long grain rice
2 tablespoons vegetable oil
1 small onion, chopped
1 garlic clove, minced
1/2 teaspoon salt-free seasoning
  blend
2 large tomatoes, peeled and
  chopped
1 cup water
1 cup low-sodium chicken broth
1/3 cup frozen peas, thawed
1/3 cup diced cooked carrots

In a large nonstick skillet over medium heat, saute rice in hot oil until lightly browned. Add the onion, garlic and seasoning blend; cook over low heat until onion is tender. Add tomatoes; cook over medium heat until softened. Add water; cover and simmer until water is absorbed. Stir in broth, peas and carrots; cover and simmer until liquid is absorbed and rice is tender, about 10 minutes. **Yield:** 6 servings.

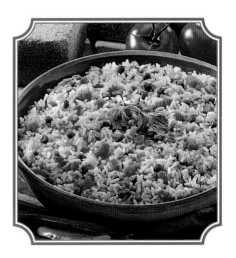

Exchanges: 1-1/2 Starch, 1 Vegetable, 1 Fat

Nutritional Information

Serving Size: 3/4 cup
Calories: 191
Sodium: 37 mg
Cholesterol: trace

Carbohydrate: 32 gm
Protein: 4 gm
Fat: 5 gm
Fiber: 2 gm

Broiled Red Potatoes

Mary Favatella Becker, Mohnton, Pennsylvania

My husband is a typical meat-and-potatoes man. Tired of the usual mashed or baked potato treatment, I began to experiment in the kitchen, and this recipe is the result.

2 unpeeled medium red potatoes
1 tablespoon margarine
1 teaspoon Worcestershire sauce
1/2 teaspoon salt-free seasoning
**   blend**
1/8 teaspoon pepper

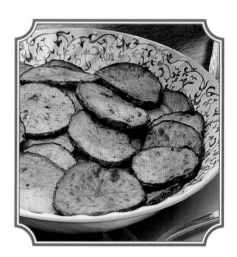

Cut potatoes into 1/4-in. slices; place in a microwave-safe bowl. Combine remaining ingredients; pour over potatoes. Cover and cook on high for 1-2 minutes or until margarine melts. Place potatoes in a single layer on a baking sheet coated with non-stick cooking spray. Broil for 5-6 minutes on each side or until browned. **Yield:** 2 servings. **Editor's Note:** This recipe was tested in a 700-watt microwave.

Exchanges: 1 Starch, 1 Fat

Nutritional Information

Serving Size: 1/2 recipe
Calories: 147
Sodium: 83 mg
Cholesterol: 0 mg

Carbohydrate: 26 gm
Protein: 4 gm
Fat: 5 gm
Fiber: 3 gm

Herbed Green Beans

Bernice Morris, Marshfield, Missouri

*When my garden is blooming with green beans and herbs,
my family can be sure I'll be reaching for
this recipe. They love this nicely seasoned side dish.*

1-1/2 pounds fresh *or* frozen green beans
1/2 cup finely chopped onion
1 tablespoon margarine
3 tablespoons lemon juice
1 tablespoon chopped fresh parsley
1-1/2 teaspoons chopped fresh thyme *or* 1/2 teaspoon dried thyme
1 teaspoon salt-free seasoning blend
1/4 teaspoon paprika

In a saucepan, cover beans with water; cook until crisp-tender. Meanwhile, in a nonstick skillet, saute onion in margarine until tender. Add lemon juice, parsley, thyme, seasoning blend and paprika. Drain beans; add to skillet and stir to coat. Serve immediately. **Yield:** 6 servings.

STAY AWAY FROM STEMS? Parsley stems are quite tender. So don't think you need to meticulously cut away parsley leaves from the stems before chopping. A few stem pieces won't be noticeable.

Exchanges: 1-1/2 Vegetable

Nutritional Information

Serving Size: 1/6 recipe
Calories: 52
Sodium: 27 mg
Cholesterol: 0 mg

Carbohydrate: 9 gm
Protein: 2 gm
Fat: 2 gm
Fiber: 1 gm

Corn-Stuffed Tomatoes

Mrs. Patrick Dore, Burlington, Ontario

My husband and I look forward to this easy, fresh-tasting side dish in summer when tomatoes are at their best. I love to invite friends over for dinner and serve these colorful tomatoes.

6 large tomatoes
1/2 cup plain bread crumbs
2 cups frozen corn, thawed
2 tablespoons *each* chopped green pepper, celery and onion
2 tablespoons half-and-half cream
1 tablespoon margarine, melted
2 tablespoons shredded reduced-fat mozzarella cheese
1/4 cup water

Cut a thin slice off the top of each tomato; scoop out and discard pulp. Invert on paper towel to drain. Combine bread crumbs, corn, green pepper, celery, onion, cream and margarine; spoon into the tomatoes. Place in an ungreased 13-in. x 9-in. x 2-in. baking dish. Sprinkle with cheese. Pour water into the baking dish. Bake, uncovered, at 350° for 30 minutes or until tomatoes are tender. **Yield:** 6 servings.

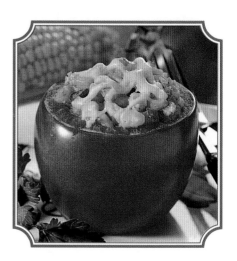

Exchanges: 2 Vegetable, 1 Starch, 1/2 Fat

Nutritional Information

Serving Size: 1/6 recipe
Calories: 153
Sodium: 130 mg
Cholesterol: 4 mg

Carbohydrate: 27 gm
Protein: 5 gm
Fat: 4 gm
Fiber: 4 gm

Wild Rice and Squash Pilaf

Erica Ollmann, San Diego, California

This pilaf is fantastic with fish or poultry and especially compatible with turkey. Since it's so colorful, I like to think it makes my turkey "dressed for the holidays".

1-1/2 cups sliced fresh mushrooms
1-1/2 cups diced peeled winter squash
   2 medium onions, finely chopped
1/2 cup chopped green pepper
   3 garlic cloves, minced
   2 tablespoons olive *or* vegetable
     oil
   3 cups cooked wild rice
1/2 cup low-sodium chicken broth
   1 tablespoon light soy sauce
1/2 teaspoon dried savory
1/4 cup sliced almonds, toasted

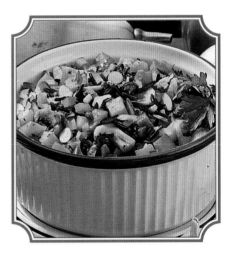

In a large saucepan, saute mushrooms, squash, onions, green pepper and garlic in oil until crisp-tender, about 5-6 minutes. Stir in the rice. Add broth, soy sauce and savory. Cover and simmer for 13-15 minutes or until squash is tender. Toss with almonds. **Yield:** 10 servings.

Exchanges: 1 Starch, 1 Vegetable, 1/2 Fat

Nutritional Information

Serving Size: 1/2 cup
Calories: 115
Sodium: 99 mg
Cholesterol: trace

Carbohydrate: 17 gm
Protein: 4 gm
Fat: 4 gm
Fiber: 2 gm

Turnips, Taters and Ham

Evelyn Thompson, Middlesboro, Kentucky

*Every year, my husband clears space in the garden to plant turnips.
He likes to eat them right out of the garden or in a
variety of dishes, including this one I created just for him.*

1 small onion, chopped
2 tablespoons reduced-fat
  margarine
2 tablespoons all-purpose flour
1/2 teaspoon salt-free seasoning
  blend
1/4 teaspoon dried basil
Dash pepper
1 cup water
1/4 cup skim milk
  4 medium potatoes, peeled and
  sliced 1/4 inch thick
  3 small turnips, peeled and sliced
  1/8 inch thick
  1 cup cubed fully cooked low-
  sodium ham
  3 tablespoons minced fresh
  parsley

In a saucepan, saute onion in margarine until tender. Stir in flour, seasoning blend, basil and pepper. Gradually stir in water and milk. Bring to a boil over medium heat; boil for 2 minutes, stirring constantly. Remove from the heat. In an 11-in. x 7-in. x 2-in. baking dish coated with non-stick cooking spray, layer potatoes, turnips and ham; pour sauce over all. Cover and bake at 350° for 1-1/4 hours or until potatoes are tender. Garnish with parsley. **Yield:** 6 servings.

Exchanges: 1 Starch, 1 Very Lean Meat, 1 Vegetable, 1/2 Fat

Nutritional Information

Serving Size: 1/6 recipe
Calories: 177
Sodium: 446 mg
Cholesterol: 20 mg

Carbohydrate: 26 gm
Protein: 12 gm
Fat: 4 gm
Fiber: 4 gm

Dilled Zucchini

Sundra Lewis, Bogalusa, Louisiana

*These super squash couldn't be easier to prepare,
and their mild flavor goes so well with chicken. I often rely on
this recipe when I have a bumper crop of zucchini to use up.*

**3 medium zucchini, halved
lengthwise
1 tablespoon margarine, melted
1/4 teaspoon dill weed
1/4 teaspoon salt-free seasoning
blend
Pepper to taste**

Place zucchini in a skillet and cover with water; bring to a boil over medium heat. Cook until tender, about 12-14 minutes. Drain; brush with margarine. Sprinkle with dill, seasoning blend and pepper. **Yield:** 6 servings.

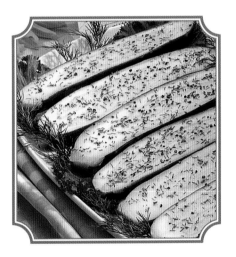

Exchanges: Free Food

Nutritional Information

Serving Size: 1/6 recipe
Calories: 18
Sodium: 19 mg
Cholesterol: 0 mg

Carbohydrate: trace
Protein: trace
Fat: 2 gm
Fiber: trace

Sesame Broccoli

Doris Heath, Bryson City, North Carolina

With a coating of tongue-tingling sauce and topping of crunchy sesame seeds, broccoli makes a fancy but fuss-free side dish. This vegetable is so nutritious that it's great to have a special way to serve it.

**1 package (10 ounces) frozen
  broccoli spears
1 tablespoon vegetable oil
1 tablespoon light soy sauce
Sugar substitute equivalent to 1
  tablespoon sugar
  2 teaspoons vinegar
  2 teaspoons sesame seeds, toasted**

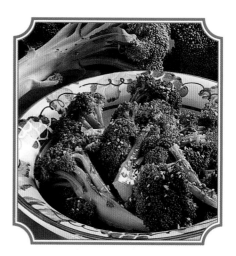

Cook broccoli according to package directions. Meanwhile, in a small saucepan, combine oil, soy sauce, sugar substitute and vinegar; heat on medium until sugar is dissolved and mixture is hot. Drain broccoli; place in a serving bowl. Drizzle with soy sauce mixture and sprinkle with sesame seeds. **Yield:** 4 servings.

Exchanges: 1/2 Vegetable, 1/2 Fat
Nutritional Information

Serving Size: 1/4 recipe
Calories: 58
Sodium: 238 mg
Cholesterol: 0 mg

Carbohydrate: 5 gm
Protein: 3 gm
Fat: 4 gm
Fiber: 3 gm

Whipped Squash

Dorothy Pritchett, Wills Point, Texas

This is an excellent way to serve a delicious vegetable—butternut squash. Its rich flavor and golden harvest color really come through in this smooth vegetable side dish.

1 butternut squash (about 2-1/2 pounds), peeled, seeded and cubed
3 cups water
3/4 teaspoon salt-free seasoning blend, *divided*
2 tablespoons margarine
Sugar substitute equivalent to 1 tablespoon sugar
1/8 to 1/4 teaspoon ground nutmeg

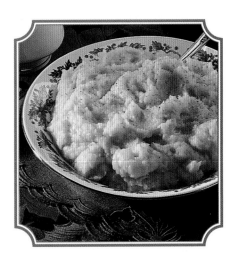

In a saucepan over medium heat, bring squash, water and 1/2 teaspoon seasoning blend to a boil. Reduce heat; cover and simmer for 20 minutes or until the squash is tender. Drain; transfer to a mixing bowl. Add margarine, sugar substitute, nutmeg and remaining seasoning blend; beat until smooth. **Yield:** 6 servings.

Exchanges: 2 Vegetable, 1/2 Starch, 1/2 Fat
Nutritional Information
Serving Size: 1/2 cup
Calories: 115
Sodium: 44 mg
Cholesterol: 0 mg

Carbohydrate: 22 gm
Protein: 2 gm
Fat: 4 gm
Fiber: 6 gm

Scalloped Turnips

Mrs. Eldon Larabee, Clearmont, Missouri

This is the only kind of cooked turnips our five grown children and 13 grandchldren will eat. The crunchy cornflake topping adds a special touch.

3 cups diced peeled turnips
2 cups water
Sugar substitute equivalent to 1 teaspoon sugar
  2 tablespoons margarine
  3 tablespoons all-purpose flour
  3/4 teaspoon salt-free seasoning blend
1-1/2 cups skim milk
  1/4 cup crushed cornflakes
  1 tablespoon chopped fresh parsley

Place the turnips, water and sugar substitute in a saucepan; simmer for 5-8 minutes or until tender. Drain and set aside. In another saucepan, melt margarine; stir in flour and seasoning blend. Gradually add milk; bring to a boil. Cook and stir for 1-2 minutes. Stir in turnips. Pour into a 1-qt. baking dish coated with nonstick cooking spray; sprinkle with cornflakes. Bake, uncovered, at 350° for 20 minutes or until bubbly. Garnish with parsley. **Yield:** 5 servings.

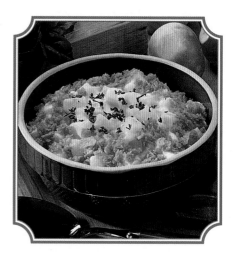

Exchanges: 1 Vegetable, 1/2 Starch, 1/2 Fat

Nutritional Information

Serving Size: 1/5 recipe
Calories: 112
Sodium: 169 mg
Cholesterol: 2 mg

Carbohydrate: 15 gm
Protein: 4 gm
Fat: 4 gm
Fiber: 2 gm

Sweet Potato Fries

Elvera Dallman, Franklin, Nebraska

Just because you're watching your waistline doesn't mean you can't indulge in some french fries. In this recipe, nutritious sweet potatoes are sprinkled with zesty seasonings and bake in the oven for a low-fat treat!

1 pound sweet potatoes
1 egg white
2 teaspoons chili powder
1/4 teaspoon garlic powder
1/4 teaspoon onion powder

Peel and cut potatoes into 1/4-in. x 1/2-in. strips. In a bowl, combine egg white and seasonings; beat well. Add potatoes; toss to coat. Place in a single layer on two baking sheets coated with nonstick cooking spray. Bake, uncovered, at 450° for 20-25 minutes or until golden brown. **Yield:** 8 servings.

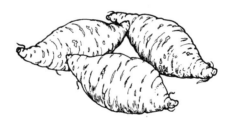

Exchanges: 1/2 Starch

Nutritional Information

Serving Size: 1/8 recipe
Calories: 54
Sodium: 43 mg
Cholesterol: 0 mg

Carbohydrate: 12 gm
Protein: 1 gm
Fat: trace
Fiber: 1 gm

Rice Medley

Doyle Rounds, Bridgewater, Virginia

*Peas, shredded carrots and seasonings dress up ordinary rice.
Your family will enjoy this tasty colorful side dish
so much they'll ask you to make it often.*

1 cup uncooked long grain rice
2-1/4 cups water
2 cups frozen peas, thawed
1 carrot, shredded
1-1/2 teaspoons salt-free herb
    seasoning blend
1 teaspoon low-sodium chicken
    bouillon granules
1 teaspoon lemon juice

In a large saucepan, combine the first six ingredients; bring to a boil. Reduce heat; cover and simmer for 15 minutes or until rice is tender. Remove from the heat; add lemon juice. Fluff with a fork. **Yield:** 10 servings.

RICE FACTS. Store uncooked white rice in an airtight container in a cool, dark place for up to 1 year. One cup uncooked long grain rice will yield about 3 cups cooked rice.

Exchanges: 1 Starch, 1/2 Vegetable

Nutritional Information

Serving Size: 1/2 cup
Calories: 96
Sodium: 48 mg
Cholesterol: trace

Carbohydrate: 20 gm
Protein: 3 gm
Fat: trace
Fiber: 2 gm

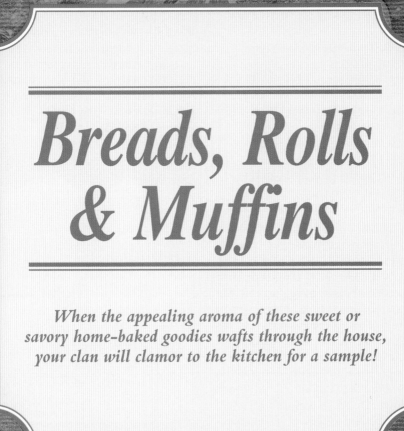

Breads, Rolls & Muffins

When the appealing aroma of these sweet or savory home-baked goodies wafts through the house, your clan will clamor to the kitchen for a sample!

Parkerhouse Rolls

Sandra Melnychenko, Grandview, Manitoba

Mom is especially well-known for these delectable golden rolls.

1 package (1/4 ounce) active dry
  yeast
6 tablespoons plus 1 teaspoon
  sugar, *divided*
1 cup warm water (110° to 115°),
  divided
1 cup warm skim milk (110° to 115°)
1 tablespoon salt
5-1/2 to 6 cups all-purpose flour
  1 egg
2 tablespoons plus 2 teaspoons
  vegetable oil
3 tablespoons margarine, melted

In a mixing bowl, dissolve yeast and 1 teaspoon sugar in 1/2 cup water; let stand for 10 minutes. Add milk, salt and remaining sugar and water. Gradually add 2 cups flour; beat until smooth. Beat in egg and oil. Stir in enough remaining flour to make a soft dough. Turn onto a floured board; knead until smooth and elastic, about 6-8 minutes. Place in a greased bowl, turning once to grease top. Cover and let rise in a warm place until doubled, about 1 hour. Punch dough down. Divide in half; roll each half on a floured board to 1/3- or 1/2-in. thickness. Cut with a floured 2-1/2-in. round cutter. Brush with margarine. Using the dull edge of a table knife, make an off-center crease in each roll. Fold along crease so the large half is on top. Press along folded edge. Place 2-3 in. apart on baking sheets coated with nonstick cooking spray. Cover and let rise until doubled, about 30 minutes. Bake at 375° for 15-20 minutes or until golden brown. Remove from pans and cool on wire racks. **Yield:** 2-1/2 dozen.

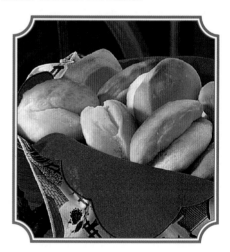

Exchanges: 1 Starch, 1/2 Fat

Nutritional Information

Serving Size: 1 roll
Calories: 120
Sodium: 253 mg
Cholesterol: 7 mg

Carbohydrate: 21 gm
Protein: 3 gm
Fat: 3 gm
Fiber: 1 gm

Wholesome Wheat Bread

Karen Wingate, Coldwater, Kansas

My sister and I were in 4-H, and Mom was our breads project leader for years. Because of that early training, fresh homemade bread like this is a staple in my own kitchen.

2 packages (1/4 ounce *each*) active dry yeast
2-1/4 cups warm water (110° to 115°)
3 tablespoons sugar
1/3 cup margarine, softened
1/3 cup honey
1/2 cup instant nonfat dry milk powder
1 tablespoon salt
4-1/2 cups whole wheat flour
2-3/4 to 3-1/2 cups all-purpose flour

In a large mixing bowl, dissolve yeast in water. Add sugar, margarine, honey, milk powder, salt and whole wheat flour; beat until smooth. Add enough all-purpose flour to form a soft dough. Turn onto a floured board; knead until smooth and elastic, about 10 minutes. Place in a greased bowl, turning once to grease top. Cover and let rise in a warm place until doubled, about 1 hour. Punch down. Shape dough into traditional loaves or divide into fourths and roll each portion into a 15-in. rope. Twist two ropes together. Place in two 9-in. x 5-in. x 3-in. loaf pans coated with nonstick cooking spray. Cover and let rise until doubled, about 30 minutes. Bake at 375° for 25-30 minutes. Remove from pans to cool on wire racks. **Yield:** 2 loaves (16 slices each).

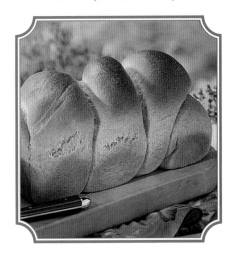

Exchanges: 1-1/2 Starch

Nutritional Information

Serving Size: 1 slice
Calories: 132
Sodium: 246 mg
Cholesterol: trace

Carbohydrate: 25 gm
Protein: 4 gm
Fat: 2 gm
Fiber: 2 gm

Corn Bread Muffins

Louise Rowe, Piqua, Ohio

I've worked in a cafeteria for over 20 years. I have come across quite a few corn bread recipes, and these muffins are some of the best I've ever tasted.

1-1/2 cups cornmeal
1/2 cup all-purpose flour
2 tablespoons sugar
2 teaspoons baking powder
1/2 teaspoon baking soda
1/2 teaspoon salt
1-1/4 cups skim buttermilk
1/4 cup unsweetened applesauce
2 egg whites
2 tablespoons vegetable oil

In a large bowl, combine the first six ingredients. Combine buttermilk, applesauce, egg whites and oil; stir into the dry ingredients just until moistened. Fill muffin cups coated with nonstick spray two-thirds full. Bake at 400° for 18-20 minutes or until muffins test done. Cool in pan 10 minutes before removing to a wire rack. **Yield:** 1 dozen.

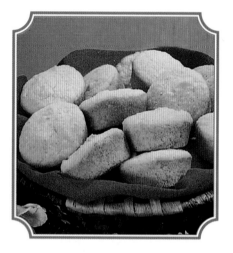

Exchanges: 1 Starch, 1/2 Fat

Nutritional Information

Serving Size: 1 muffin
Calories: 126
Sodium: 225 mg
Cholesterol: 1 mg

Carbohydrate: 21 gm
Protein: 3 gm
Fat: 3 gm
Fiber: 1 gm

Cinnamon Rolls

Kim Marie VanRheenan, Mendota, Illinois

This recipe is simplified by starting with frozen bread dough.
Chopped apple contributes to the texture and taste.
I like to surprise my family with these rolls on weekend mornings.

1 loaf (1 pound) frozen white bread dough, thawed
2 tablespoons reduced-fat margarine, softened
1 tablespoon ground cinnamon
1 small tart apple, peeled and chopped
3/4 cup raisins
1/2 cup chopped pecans

Roll dough into a 12-in. x 9-in. rectangle. Brush with margarine; sprinkle with cinnamon. Sprinkle the apple, raisins and pecans evenly over dough. Roll up, jelly roll style, starting at a long side. Cut into 12 slices, 1 in. each. Place rolls, cut side down, in an 11-in. x 7-in. x 2-in. baking dish coated with nonstick cooking spray. Cover and let rise until doubled, about 1 hour. Bake at 350° for 25-30 minutes or until golden brown. Cool on a wire rack. **Yield:** 1 dozen.

SLICING CINNAMON ROLLS. Instead of slicing cinnamon rolls with a knife, try using dental floss. Place a piece of floss under the rolled dough, 1-inch from the end. Bring the sides of the floss up around dough and cross it over at the top, cutting through the dough and filling. Repeat at 1-inch intervals.

Exchanges: 1-1/2 Starch, 1/2 Fruit, 1/2 Fat

Nutritional Information

Serving Size: 1 roll	Carbohydrate: 29 gm
Calories: 180	Protein: 5 gm
Sodium: 235 mg	Fat: 6 gm
Cholesterol: 0 mg	Fiber: 2 gm

Onion Zucchini Bread

Annie Sassard, Ft. McCoy, Florida

*Only two steps and this bread is mixed and ready for the oven!
You'll love the flavor of onion and Parmesan cheese. Baked in a round pan,
it looks nice on the table whole or sliced in wedges.*

3 cups all-purpose flour
3/4 cup chopped onion
1/4 cup grated Parmesan cheese,
    divided
4 teaspoons baking powder
1/2 teaspoon salt
1/2 teaspoon baking soda
1 cup skim buttermilk
1/4 cup vegetable oil
Egg substitute equivalent to 2 eggs
3/4 cup finely shredded zucchini

In a bowl, combine flour, onion, 2 tablespoons of Parmesan cheese, baking powder, salt and baking soda. In a small bowl, mix buttermilk, oil, egg substitute and zucchini; stir into flour mixture just until blended. Spoon into a 9-in. round baking pan coated with nonstick coating spray.

Sprinkle with remaining Parmesan. Bake at 350° for 40 minutes. **Yield:** 8 servings.

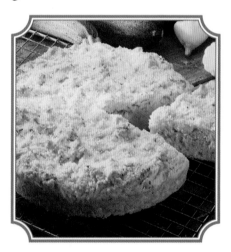

Exchanges: 2 Starch, 1-1/2 Fat, 1/2 Vegetable
Nutritional Information

Serving Size: 1/8 recipe
Calories: 281
Sodium: 448 mg
Cholesterol: 4 mg

Carbohydrate: 40 gm
Protein: 8 gm
Fat: 9 gm
Fiber: 2 gm

Pumpkin Date Bread

Ruth McKay, Hopkins, Minnesota

I appreciate recipes that fit my husband's restricted diet. Pumpkin makes this sweet bread nice and moist, while seasonings add flavor.

1/3 cup margarine, softened
3 tablespoons brown sugar
Egg substitute equivalent to 2 eggs
1 cup cooked *or* canned pumpkin
1 cup whole wheat flour
1/2 cup all-purpose flour
1 teaspoon baking powder
1 teaspoon baking soda
1-1/2 teaspoons ground cinnamon
1/2 teaspoon ground nutmeg
1/4 teaspoon salt
1/4 teaspoon ground cloves
1/4 teaspoon ground allspice
1/2 cup buttermilk
1 cup quick-cooking oats
1/2 cup chopped dates

In a mixing bowl, cream margarine and brown sugar. Beat in egg substitute and pumpkin. Combine the dry ingredients; add to creamed mixture alternately with buttermilk. Stir in oats and dates. Pour into an 8-in. x 4-in. x 2-in. loaf pan coated with nonstick cooking spray. Bake at 350° for 75 minutes or until a toothpick inserted near the center comes out clean. Cool in pan 10 minutes; remove to a wire rack to cool. **Yield:** 1 loaf (15 slices).

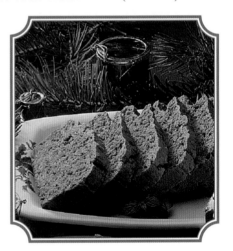

Exchanges: 1 Starch, 1 Fat

Nutritional Information

Serving Size: 1 slice
Calories: 137
Sodium: 197 mg
Cholesterol: trace

Carbohydrate: 21 gm
Protein: 4 gm
Fat: 5 gm
Fiber: 3 gm

Healthy Wheat Bread

Betty Howell, Wichita, Kansas

*This tasty bread has a slightly sweet flavor.
I developed the recipe to suit my husband's diet.*

3 to 4 cups all-purpose flour,
divided
2 teaspoons salt
**2 packages (1/4 ounce *each*) active
dry yeast**
1 cup water
1/2 cup honey
2 tablespoons vegetable oil
1 cup low-fat cottage cheese
4 egg whites
1-1/2 cups whole wheat flour
1/2 cup wheat germ
1/2 cup old-fashioned oats

In a mixing bowl, combine 2 cups all-purpose flour, salt and yeast. In a saucepan, heat water, honey and oil to 120°-130°; stir in cottage cheese. Add to flour mixture with egg whites; blend on low until moistened. Beat for 3 minutes on medium. Add whole wheat flour, wheat germ, oats and enough of the remaining all-purpose flour to form a soft dough. Turn onto a floured surface; knead until smooth and elastic, about 6-8 minutes. Place in a greased bowl, turning once to grease top.

Cover and let rise in a warm place until doubled, about 1 hour. Punch dough down. Shape into two loaves. Place in two 8-in. x 4-in. x 2-in. loaf pans coated with nonstick cooking spray. Cover and let rise until doubled, about 1 hour. Bake at 375° for 35-40 minutes or until golden brown; cover with foil during the last 15 minutes to prevent overbrowning. Remove from pans; cool on wire racks. **Yield:** 2 loaves (16 slices each).

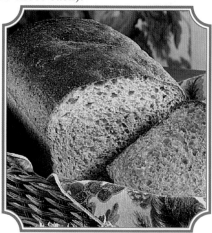

Exchanges: 1-1/4 Starch

Nutritional Information

Serving Size: 1 slice
Calories: 106
Sodium: 180 mg
Cholesterol: 1 mg

Carbohydrate: 20 gm
Protein: 4 gm
Fat: 2 gm
Fiber: 2 gm

Early-Riser Muffins

Brenda Offutt, Lincoln, Nebraska

Despite the name, you don't have to be an early-riser to enjoy these hearty muffins (we often make them for brunch). My husband and children come running when they smell these tender muffins baking.

2 cups all-purpose flour
2 tablespoons sugar
1 tablespoon baking powder
1/4 teaspoon salt
1/4 teaspoon ground mustard
Egg substitute equivalent to 1 egg
1 cup skim milk
1/3 cup margarine, melted
3/4 cup finely chopped low-sodium ham
1/2 cup shredded reduced-fat cheddar cheese

In a bowl, combine flour, sugar, baking powder, salt and mustard. Combine egg substitute, milk and margarine; stir into dry ingredients just until moistened. Fold in ham and cheese. Fill muffin cups coated with nonstick cooking spray two-thirds full. Bake at 400° for 20-25 minutes or until muffins test done. Cool in pan 10 minutes before removing to a wire rack. **Yield:** 1 dozen.

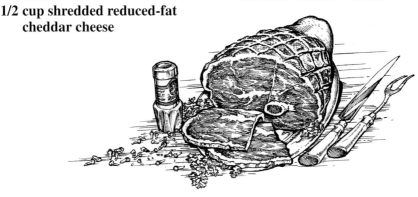

Exchanges: 1 Starch, 1 Lean Meat, 1 Fat

Nutritional Information

Serving Size: 1 muffin
Calories: 189
Sodium: 480 mg
Cholesterol: 17 mg
Carbohydrate: 20 gm
Protein: 11 gm
Fat: 7 gm
Fiber: trace

Skillet Herb Bread

Shirley Smith, Yorba Linda, California

*My mother, grandmother and aunts had their own specialty
when it came to bread, but Mom's was my favorite.
The flavors call to mind the taste of corn bread stuffing*

1-1/2 cups all-purpose flour
2 tablespoons sugar
4 teaspoons baking powder
1-1/2 teaspoons salt
1 teaspoon rubbed sage
1 teaspoon dried thyme
1-1/2 cups cornmeal
1-1/2 cups chopped celery
1 cup chopped onion
**1 jar (2 ounces) diced
    pimientos, drained**
Egg substitute equivalent to 3 eggs
1-1/2 cups skim milk
1/3 cup vegetable oil

In a large bowl, combine the flour, sugar,
baking powder, salt, sage and thyme.
Combine cornmeal, celery, onion and
pimientos; add to dry ingredients and mix
well. Add egg substitute, milk and oil; stir
just until moistened. Pour into a 10- or 11-
in. ovenproof skillet coated with nonstick cooking spray. Bake at 400° for 35-
45 minutes or until bread tests done. Serve
warm. **Yield:** 10 servings.

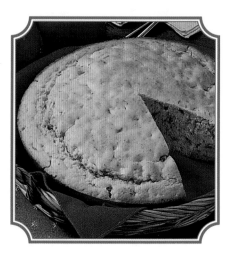

Exchanges: 2 Starch, 1-1/2 Fat, 1/2 Vegetable

Nutritional Information

Serving Size: 1/10 recipe
Calories: 266
Sodium: 521 mg
Cholesterol: 1 mg

Carbohydrate: 39 gm
Protein: 7 gm
Fat: 9 gm
Fiber: 3 gm

Broccoli Muffins

Theresa Rentfro, Cedar Creek, Texas

Because my family loves muffins, I'm always on the lookout for new variations. When I tried these nutritional muffins the first time, they were a hit and became a favorite addition to our family meals.

1-3/4 cups all-purpose flour
1 cup quick-cooking oats
1/4 cup sugar
2 teaspoons baking powder
1/4 teaspoon salt
1 cup skim milk
1/3 cup vegetable oil
Egg substitute equivalent to 1 egg
1 cup chopped fresh broccoli, blanched
1/2 cup shredded reduced-fat cheddar cheese

In a large bowl, combine flour, oats, sugar, baking powder and salt. In a small bowl, mix milk, oil and egg substitute; stir into dry ingredients just until moistened. Fold in broccoli and cheese. Spoon into muffin cups coated with nonstick cooking spray. Bake at 400° for 18-20 minutes or until top springs back when lightly touched. **Yield:** 1 dozen.

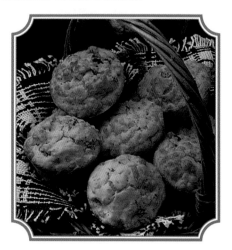

Exchanges: 1-1/2 Starch, 1 Fat

Nutritional Information

Serving Size: 1 muffin
Calories: 181
Sodium: 129 mg
Cholesterol: 1 mg

Carbohydrate: 23 gm
Protein: 5 gm
Fat: 8 gm
Fiber: 1 gm

Fruit 'n' Nut Loaf

Janet Boulger, Botwood, Newfoundland

I enjoy all kinds of cooking, but I especially like baking delicious breads like this! It's chock-full of good things like apricots, almonds and bananas.

1 cup all-purpose flour
1 cup whole wheat flour
1 cup raisins
2/3 cup instant nonfat dry milk powder
1/2 cup packed brown sugar
1/2 cup finely chopped dried apricots
1/3 cup wheat germ
1/4 cup chopped toasted almonds
2 teaspoons baking powder
1/2 teaspoon baking soda
1/2 teaspoon salt
Egg substitute equivalent to 3 eggs
3/4 cup unsweetened orange juice
1/2 cup vegetable oil
1/2 cup molasses
2 large ripe bananas, mashed (about 1-1/3 cups)

In a large bowl, combine the first 11 ingredients. In another bowl, beat the egg substitute, juice, oil, molasses and bananas; stir into dry ingredients just until moistened. Pour into two 8-in. x 4-in. x 2-in. loaf pans coated with nonstick cooking spray. Bake at 325° for 1 hour or until bread tests done. Cool for 10 minutes; remove from pans to wire racks to cool. **Yield:** 2 loaves (14 slices each).

Exchanges: 1 Starch, 1 Fat, 1/2 Fruit

Nutritional Information

Serving Size: 1 slice
Calories: 155
Sodium: 109 mg
Cholesterol: trace

Carbohydrate: 25 gm
Protein: 3 gm
Fat: 5 gm
Fiber: 2 gm

Dad's Flat Bread

Anne Heinonen, Howell, Michigan

There's no mistaking that this flavorful bread is homemade.
It has a wonderful texture and lovely golden color.
Dad enjoyed making this bread for the family.

1 package (1/4 ounce) active
   dry yeast
2 cups warm water (110° to
   115°), *divided*
1/3 cup sugar
2 tablespoons vegetable oil
1 tablespoon salt
1/2 cup rye *or* whole wheat flour
5-1/2 to 6 cups all-purpose flour

In a large mixing bowl, dissolve yeast in 1/2 cup of water. Add sugar, oil, salt, rye or whole wheat flour, 3 cups all-purpose flour and remaining water; beat until smooth. Add enough remaining all-purpose flour to form a soft dough. Turn onto a floured board; knead until smooth and elastic, about 6-8 minutes. Place in a greased bowl, turning once to grease top. Cover and let rise in a warm place until doubled, about 1 hour. Punch dough down. Divide in half. On a baking sheet coated with nonstick cooking spray, flatten each half to 1-in. thickness. Pierce each loaf several times with a fork. Cover and let rise in a warm place until nearly doubled, about 30 minutes. Bake at 375° for 25-30 minutes or until golden brown. **Yield:** 2 loaves (16 slices each).

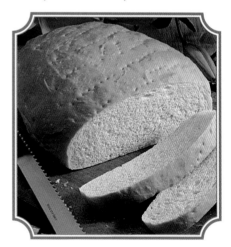

Exchanges: 1-1/4 Starch

Nutritional Information

Serving Size: 1 slice
Calories: 100
Sodium: 221 mg
Cholesterol: 0 mg

Carbohydrate: 20 gm
Protein: 2 gm
Fat: 1 gm
Fiber: 1 gm

Cheesy Italian Bread

Cookie Curci-Wright, San Jose, California

This crusty bread is always a big treat. It goes so well with an Italian meal or alongside a big bowl of soup.

1 package (1/4 ounce) active dry
   yeast
1-1/4 cups warm water (110° to 115°)
2 tablespoons sugar
1 teaspoon salt
1 teaspoon garlic salt
1/2 cup grated Romano cheese
3 to 3-1/2 cups all-purpose flour
1 tablespoon cornmeal

In a mixing bowl, dissolve yeast in water. Add sugar, salt, garlic salt, cheese and 2 cups of flour; beat until smooth. Add enough remaining flour to form a soft dough. Turn onto a floured surface; knead until smooth and elastic, about 6-8 minutes. Place in a greased bowl, turning once to grease top. Cover and let rise in a warm place until doubled, about 1 hour. Punch dough down; divide in half. Shape each half into a 14-in. loaf. Place on an ungreased baking sheet sprinkled with cornmeal. Cover and let rise until doubled, about 45 minutes. Brush loaves with water. Make three diagonal slashes about 1/2 in. deep with a very sharp knife in each loaf. Fill a 13-in. x 9-in. x 2-in. baking pan with 1 in. of hot water and place on the bottom oven rack. Bake loaves at 400° for 20-25 minutes. Remove to wire racks. **Yield:** 2 loaves (16 slices each).

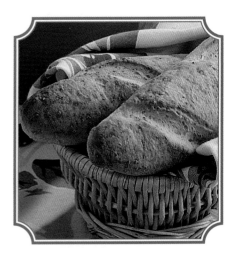

Exchanges: 1/2 Starch
Nutritional Information

Serving Size: 1 slice
Calories: 53
Sodium: 149 mg
Cholesterol: 2 mg

Carbohydrate: 10 gm
Protein: 2 gm
Fat: 1 gm
Fiber: trace

Oat-Bran Bread

Wanda Cutler, Canby, Oregon

I was a novice at bread baking when a neighbor gave me this recipe. I've been baking bread for years and still rely on this tried-and-true recipe.

2 packages (1/4 ounce *each*) active dry yeast
4-1/2 cups warm water (110° to 115°), *divided*
3/4 cup vegetable oil
3/4 cup sugar
1/4 cup molasses
2 teaspoons salt
1/4 cup wheat germ
1/4 cup oat bran
2 cups quick-cooking oats
3 cups whole wheat flour
7 to 7-1/2 cups all-purpose flour

In a large mixing bowl, dissolve yeast in 1/2 cup warm water. Add oil, sugar, molasses, salt, wheat germ, bran and remaining warm water; mix well. Add oats, whole wheat flour and 2 cups all-purpose flour; beat until smooth. Add enough remaining all-purpose flour to form a soft dough. Turn onto a floured board; knead until smooth and elastic, about 6-8 minutes. Place in a greased bowl, turning once to grease top. Cover and let rise in a warm place until doubled, about 1 hour. Punch dough down and shape into four loaves. Place in four 8-in. x 4-in. x 2-in. loaf pans coated with nonstick cooking spray. Cover and let rise until doubled, about 30 minutes. Bake at 350° for 30-35 minutes. Remove from pans and cool on wire racks. **Yield:** 4 loaves (16 slices each).

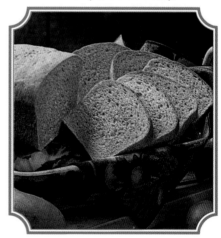

Exchanges: 1 Starch, 1/2 Fat

Nutritional Information

Serving Size: 1 slice
Calories: 117
Sodium: 75 mg
Cholesterol: 0 mg

Carbohydrate: 20 gm
Protein: 3 gm
Fat: 3 gm
Fiber: 1 gm

Blue-Ribbon Herb Rolls

Mary Ann Evans, Tarpon Springs, Florida

I developed this recipe by using several ideas and techniques while learning the art of bread making. It won a blue ribbon at our county fair.

2 packages (1/4 ounce *each*)
   active dry yeast
2-3/4 cups warm water (110° to
   115°), *divided*
1 egg, beaten
1/3 cup vegetable oil
1/4 cup honey *or* molasses
1 tablespoon salt
2 teaspoons dill weed
2 teaspoons dried thyme
2 teaspoons dried basil
1 teaspoon onion powder
4 cups whole wheat flour
4 to 4-1/2 cups all-purpose
   flour

In a mixing bowl, dissolve yeast in 1/2 cup warm water. Add the next nine ingredients and remaining water; beat until smooth. Gradually add enough all-purpose flour to form a soft dough. Turn onto a floured board; knead until smooth and elastic, 6-8 minutes. Place in a greased bowl; turn once to grease top. Cover and let rise in a warm place until doubled, about 1 hour. Punch dough down. Shape into 1-in. balls. Place three balls each in muffin cups coated with nonstick cooking spray. Cover and let rise until doubled, 20-25 minutes. Bake at 375° for 12-15 minutes or until tops are golden brown. Remove to a wire rack. **Yield:** 4 dozen.

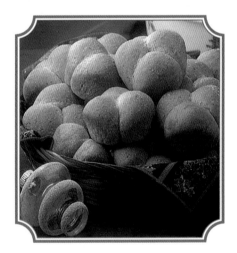

Exchanges: 1 Starch, 1/4 Fat
Nutritional Information

Serving Size: 1 roll
Calories: 93
Sodium: 149 mg
Cholesterol: 4 mg

Carbohydrate: 17 gm
Protein: 3 gm
Fat: 2 gm
Fiber: 2 gm

English Muffin Bread

Donna Meyer, Dayton, Ohio

You can bake this bread either in clean coffee cans for a change of pace or regular loaf pans. This bread is really delicious when toasted.

6 cups all-purpose flour,
  divided
2 packages (1/4 ounce *each*)
  active dry yeast
1 tablespoon sugar
2 teaspoons salt
1/4 teaspoon baking soda
2 cups warm skim milk
  (120° to 130°)
1/2 cup warm water (120° to 130°)
2 tablespoons cornmeal

In a bowl, combine 3 cups flour, yeast, sugar, salt and baking soda. Stir in milk and water; mix well. Stir in remaining flour (batter will be soft). Do not knead. Spray three 13-oz. coffee cans or 8-in. x 4-in. x 2-in. loaf pans with nonstick cooking spray. Sprinkle with cornmeal. Spoon batter into pans; sprinkle cornmeal on top. Cover and let rise in a warm place until doubled, about 45 minutes. Bake at 400° for 20-25 minutes or until golden brown. Remove from pans to cool on wire racks. **Yield:** 3 loaves (16 slices each).

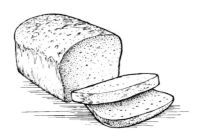

Exchanges: 3/4 Starch
Nutritional Information

Serving Size: 1 slice
Calories: 64
Sodium: 110 mg
Cholesterol: trace

Carbohydrate: 13 gm
Protein: 2 gm
Fat: trace
Fiber: 1 gm

Sunny Cornmeal Muffins

Lethea Weber, Newport, Arkansas

Most muffin recipes make such a big batch that I can't possibly eat them all. So I was thrilled to find this recipe that makes just two muffins.

1/4 cup reduced-fat biscuit/baking mix
1/4 cup cornmeal
1 tablespoon sugar
1/4 cup skim milk
Egg substitute equivalent to 1 egg
2 teaspoons vegetable oil

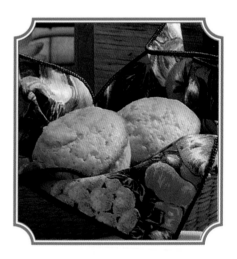

In a small bowl, combine the baking mix, cornmeal and sugar. Combine milk, egg substitute and oil; stir into dry ingredients just until moistened (batter will be thin). Pour into two 6-oz. ovenproof custard cups coated with nonstick cooking spray. Bake at 400° for 15-18 minutes or until golden brown. **Yield:** 2 muffins. **Editor's Note:** Muffins may be baked in a muffin pan; fill empty cups halfway with water.

Exchanges: 1-1/2 Starch, 1-1/2 Fat, 1/2 Lean Meat

Nutritional Information

Serving Size: 1 muffin
Calories: 243
Sodium: 251 mg
Cholesterol: 1 mg

Carbohydrate: 33 gm
Protein: 7 gm
Fat: 9 gm
Fiber: 1 gm

Oatmeal Wheat Bread

Jackie Gavin, Essex Junction, Vermont

My mother taught me to make this bread when I was 10 years old. It tastes marvelous and it's good for you.

1-3/4 cups boiling water
   1 cup quick-cooking oats
   1/2 cup molasses
   1/4 cup shortening
   1/4 cup orange juice
1-1/2 teaspoons salt
   2 packages (1/4 ounce *each*) active
    dry yeast
   1/2 cup warm water (110° to 115°)
2-1/2 cups whole wheat flour
   3 to 3-1/2 cups all-purpose flour
   1 tablespoon margarine, melted

In a large mixing bowl, combine boiling water, oats, molasses, shortening, orange juice and salt; let stand until warm (110°-115°). In a small bowl, dissolve yeast in warm water; add to oat mixture. Add whole wheat flour and beat until smooth. Add enough all-purpose flour to form a soft dough. Turn onto a floured board; knead until smooth and elastic, about 6-8 minutes. Place in a greased bowl, turning once to grease top. Cover and let rise in a warm place until doubled, about 1 hour. Punch dough down. Shape into two loaves; place in two 8-in. x 4-in. x 2-in. loaf pans coated with nonstick cooking spray. Cover and let rise until doubled, about 45 minutes. Bake at 350° for 40 minutes. Remove from pans; brush with margarine. Cool on wire racks. **Yield:** 2 loaves (16 slices each).

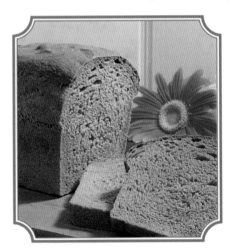

Exchanges: 1 Starch, 1/2 Fat

Nutritional Information

Serving Size: 1 slice
Calories: 117
Sodium: 116 mg
Cholesterol: 0 mg

Carbohydrate: 21 gm
Protein: 3 gm
Fat: 2 gm
Fiber: 2 gm

Dilly Parmesan Bread

Marian Bell, Cedar Grove, New Jersey

This recipe originally called for chives. Over the years, I've substituted dill with taste-tempting results.

2 packages (1/4 ounce *each*) active
   dry yeast
2 cups warm water (110° to 115°)
4 to 4-1/2 cups all-purpose flour
1/2 cup grated Parmesan cheese
2 tablespoons sugar
2 tablespoons dill weed
2 tablespoons margarine, softened
2 teaspoons salt
TOPPING:
   2 tablespoons grated Parmesan
   cheese
1 teaspoon margarine, melted

In a mixing bowl, dissolve yeast in water. Add 3 cups of flour, Parmesan cheese, sugar, dill, margarine and salt; beat until smooth, about 2 minutes. Gradually beat in remaining flour (do not knead). Place in a greased bowl; turn once to grease top. Cover and let rise in a warm place until doubled, about 45 minutes. Stir batter down and beat 25 strokes with a spoon. Place in a 9-in. springform pan coated with nonstick cooking spray (do not allow to rise). Sprinkle with Parmesan cheese. Bake at 375° for 55-60 minutes or until golden brown. Brush with margarine. Remove from pan and cool on a wire rack. **Yield:** 1 loaf (16 slices).

Exchanges: 1-1/2 Starch, 1/2 Fat

Nutritional Information

Serving Size: 1 slice
Calories: 153
Sodium: 383 mg
Cholesterol: 3 mg

Carbohydrate: 26 gm
Protein: 5 gm
Fat: 3 gm
Fiber: 1 gm

Oatmeal Dinner Rolls

Patricia Staudt, Marble Rock, Iowa

These fluffy rolls go perfectly with any meal. They have a delicious homemade flavor that's irresistible. They're not hard to make, and they bake up nice and high.

2 cups water
1 cup quick-cooking oats
3 tablespoons margarine
1 package (1/4 ounce) active
  dry yeast
1/3 cup warm water (110° to 115°)
1/3 cup packed brown sugar
1 tablespoon sugar
1-1/2 teaspoons salt
4-3/4 to 5-1/4 cups all-purpose flour

In a saucepan, bring water to a boil; add oats and margarine. Cook and stir for 1 minute. Remove from the heat; cool to lukewarm. In a mixing bowl, dissolve yeast in warm water. Add the oat mixture, sugars, salt and 4 cups of flour; beat until smooth. Add enough remaining flour to form a soft dough. Turn onto a floured board; knead until smooth and elastic, about 6-8 minutes. Place in a greased bowl, turning once to grease top. Cover and let rise in a warm place until doubled, about 1 hour. Punch dough down; allow to rest for 10 minutes. Shape into 18 balls. Place in two 9-in. round baking pans coated with nonstick cooking spray. Cover and let rise until doubled, about 45 minutes. Bake at 350° for 20-25 minutes or until golden brown. Remove from pan to wire racks. **Yield:** 1-1/2 dozen.

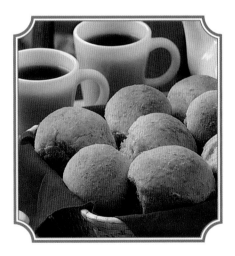

Exchanges: 1-1/2 Starch, 1/2 Fat

Nutritional Information

Serving Size: 1 roll
Calories: 172
Sodium: 216 mg
Cholesterol: 0 mg

Carbohydrate: 33 gm
Protein: 4 gm
Fat: 2 gm
Fiber: 1 gm

Yogurt Herb Bread

Carol Forcum, Marion, Illinois

Slices from these high, savory loaves always seem to vanish quickly from a buffet. An enticing combination of herbs makes a distinctive flavor folks rave about.

5-1/2 to 6-1/2 cups all-purpose flour
  2 packages (1/4 ounce *each*) active dry yeast
  2 tablespoons sugar
  2 teaspoons salt
  1 cup water
  1 cup (8 ounces) plain nonfat yogurt
  3 tablespoons vegetable oil
  1 teaspoon dill weed
  1/2 teaspoon dried chives
  1/4 teaspoon *each* dried oregano, thyme and basil

In a large mixing bowl, combine 2-1/2 cups flour, yeast, sugar and salt. In a small saucepan, heat water and yogurt to 120°-130°. Add to flour mixture; mix well. Add oil, herbs and enough of the remaining flour to form a stiff dough. Turn onto a floured surface; knead until smooth and elastic, about 6-8 minutes. Place in a greased bowl, turning once to grease top. Cover and let rise in a warm place until doubled, about 1 hour. Punch dough down; shape into two loaves. Place in two 8-in. x 4-in. x 2-in. loaf pans coated with non-stick cooking spray. Cover and let rise until doubled, about 1 hour. Bake at 375° for 35-40 minutes or until golden brown. Remove from pans to cool on wire racks. **Yield:** 2 loaves (16 slices each).

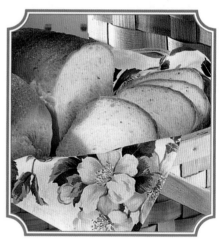

Exchanges: 1 Starch, 1/2 Fat

Nutritional Information

Serving Size: 1 slice
Calories: 98
Sodium: 153 mg
Cholesterol: trace

Carbohydrate: 18 gm
Protein: 3 gm
Fat: 2 gm
Fiber: trace

Home-Style Cheese Muffins

Mina Dyck, Boissevain, Manitoba

These muffins are a savory addition to your favorite breakfast or brunch. Your family will love them, and you can whip them up in a hurry!

2 cups all-purpose flour
3 teaspoons baking powder
1/2 teaspoon salt
1 egg, lightly beaten
1 cup skim milk
1/4 cup margarine, melted
1/2 cup shredded reduced-fat cheddar cheese

In a bowl, combine flour, baking powder and salt. Mix egg, milk and margarine; stir into dry ingredients just until moistened. Fold in cheese. Fill muffin cups coated with nonstick cooking spray two-thirds full. Bake at 400° for 20-25 minutes or until golden brown. **Yield:** 1 dozen.

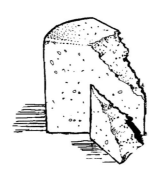

Exchanges: 1 Starch, 1 Fat

Nutritional Information

Serving Size: 1 muffin
Calories: 128
Sodium: 237 mg
Cholesterol: 19 mg

Carbohydrate: 17 gm
Protein: 5 gm
Fat: 4 gm
Fiber: trace

Whole Wheat Braids

Suella Miller, LaGrange, Indiana

*There's nothing like fresh bread to complete a meal.
I've had very good results with this recipe.
Braiding the dough makes a pretty presentation.*

**3 packages (1/4 ounce *each*)
  active dry yeast
3 cups warm water (110° to 115°)
1/2 cup sugar
3 eggs
1/3 cup vegetable oil
1 tablespoon salt
5 cups whole wheat flour
4 to 4-1/2 cups all-purpose flour**

In a mixing bowl, dissolve yeast in warm water. Add the sugar, eggs, oil, salt and whole wheat flour; beat until smooth. Add enough all-purpose flour to form a soft dough. Turn onto a floured surface; knead until smooth and elastic, about 6-8 minutes. Place in a greased bowl; turn once to grease top. Cover and let rise in a warm place until doubled, about 1 hour. Punch dough down. Divide into nine pieces; shape each piece into a 14-in. rope and braid three ropes together. Place in three 8-in. x 4-in. x 2-in. loaf pans coated with nonstick cooking spray. Cover and let rise until doubled, about 30 minutes. Bake at 350° for 40-45 minutes. Remove from pans to cool on wire racks. **Yield:** 3 loaves (16 slices each).

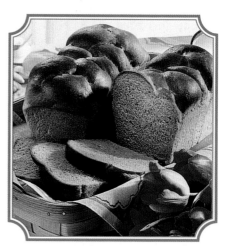

Exchanges: 1-1/2 Starch

Nutritional Information

Serving Size: 1 slice
Calories: 108
Sodium: 152 mg
Cholesterol: 13 mg

Carbohydrate: 19 gm
Protein: 3 gm
Fat: 2 gm
Fiber: 2 gm

Sweet Treats

You don't have to do without desserts on a restricted diet. These cakes, cookies, pies and more will make your mouth water without expanding your waistline!

Baked Apples

Marcia Weber, Elkhorn, Nebraska

Who says desserts have to be laden with chocolate to be delicious? In this recipe, apples are dressed up with three ingredients for a fuss-free treat.

4 medium tart apples, cored
4 teaspoons low-sugar strawberry spreadable fruit
1/2 teaspoon ground cinnamon
1-1/2 cups unsweetened orange juice

Place apples in a foil-lined 8-in. square baking pan. Spoon 1 teaspoon jam into the center of each apple; sprinkle with cinnamon. Pour orange juice into pan. Bake, uncovered, at 400° for 20-25 minutes or until apples are tender. Serve immediately. **Yield:** 4 servings.

BEST FOR BAKING. Cortland, Granny Smith, Jonathon, Newtown Pippin, Northern Spy, Rome Beauty and York Imperial are tart varieties that work well for baking. Leave the peel intact so the apple holds together better.

Exchanges: 2 Fruit

Nutritional Information

Serving Size: 1 apple
Calories: 109
Sodium: 9 mg
Cholesterol: 0 mg

Carbohydrate: 29 gm
Protein: 1 gm
Fat: trace
Fiber: 3 gm

Fresh Raspberry Pie

Patricia Staudt, Marble Rock, Iowa

Mouth-watering fresh raspberries star in this luscious pie.
There's nothing to distract from the tangy berry flavor and gorgeous ruby color.
We enjoy the taste of summer with each slice.

1/4 cup sugar
  1 tablespoon cornstarch
  1 cup water
  1 package (.3 ounce) sugar-free
    raspberry gelatin
  4 cups fresh *or* frozen raspberries,
    thawed
  1 reduced-fat graham cracker
    crust (8 inches)
1/2 cup nonfat whipped topping

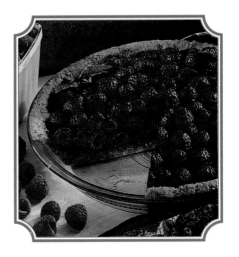

In a saucepan, combine sugar and cornstarch. Add the water and bring to a boil, stirring constantly. Cook and stir for 2 minutes. Remove from the heat; stir in gelatin until dissolved. Cool for 15 minutes. Place raspberries in the crust; slowly pour gelatin mixture over berries. Refrigerate until set, about 3 hours. Garnish with whipped topping. **Yield:** 8 servings.

Exchanges: 1 Starch, 1 Fat

Nutritional Information

Serving Size: 1 slice
Calories: 162
Sodium: 118 mg
Cholesterol: 0 mg

Carbohydrate: 31 gm
Protein: 2 gm
Fat: 1 gm
Fiber: 4 gm

Pumpkin Bundt Cake

Lucille Noyd, Shrewsbury, Massachusetts

When you tell people how easy it is to make this deliciously moist cake, they won't believe it! The secret ingredient in this treasured recipe is butterscotch pudding.

1 package (18-1/4 ounces) reduced-fat yellow cake mix
1 package (1 ounce) instant sugar-free butterscotch pudding mix
1 cup cooked *or* canned pumpkin
Egg substitute equivalent to 4 eggs
1/4 cup water
1/4 cup vegetable oil
1-1/2 to 2 teaspoons pumpkin pie spice
1 cup fat-free whipped topping

In a mixing bowl, combine the first seven ingredients. Beat on low speed for 2 minutes. Transfer to a 10-in. fluted tube pan coated with nonstick cooking spray. Bake at 350° for 35-40 minutes or until a toothpick inserted near the center comes out clean. Cool in pan for 10 minutes before removing to a wire rack. Garnish each slice with 1 tablespoon whipped topping. **Yield:** 16 servings.

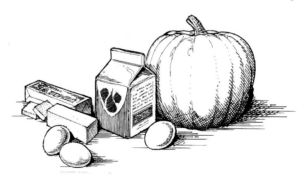

Exchanges: 2 Starch, 1/2 Fat

Nutritional Information

Serving Size: 1/16 recipe
Calories: 194
Sodium: 340 mg
Cholesterol: trace

Carbohydrate: 32 gm
Protein: 4 gm
Fat: 6 gm
Fiber: 1 gm

Pineapple Delight

Shirlye Price, Hartford, Kentucky

*I received this recipe at a meeting for diabetics many years ago.
I've shared this dessert with many friends on restricted diets.*

1 cup reduced-fat graham cracker crumbs (about 16 squares)
3 tablespoons margarine, melted
1 package (.3 ounce) sugar-free lemon gelatin
1 cup boiling water
1 carton (24 ounces) low-fat cottage cheese
Sugar substitute equivalent to 7 teaspoons sugar
2 teaspoons cornstarch
1 tablespoon water
1 can (8 ounces) unsweetened crushed pineapple, undrained

In a bowl, combine cracker crumbs and margarine. Press into an ungreased 9-in. square baking pan. Refrigerate until firm. In a bowl, combine gelatin and water; stir until dissolved. Cool to room temperature. In a blender, combine the cottage cheese and sugar substitute; cover and process until smooth. Slowly add gelatin mixture and blend until smooth. Pour into crust. Refrigerate until firm. Meanwhile, in a saucepan, combine cornstarch and water until smooth. Add pineapple. Bring to a boil. Cook and stir for 2 minutes or until thickened. Cool to room temperature. Spread over gelatin layer. Refrigerate for at least 1 hour before serving. **Yield:** 12 servings.

Exchanges: 1 Lean Meat, 1 Fruit

Nutritional Information

Serving Size: 1/12 recipe
Calories: 105
Sodium: 307 mg
Cholesterol: 5 mg

Carbohydrate: 9 gm
Protein: 8 gm
Fat: 4 gm
Fiber: trace

Low-Fat Oatmeal Cookies

Kathleen Nolan, Lawrenceville, Georgia

*These oatmeal cookies are chewy with
old-fashioned goodness. People will never know these treats
are low in fat…and you don't have to tell them!*

1 cup all-purpose flour
1 cup quick-cooking oats
1/2 cup sugar
1/2 teaspoon baking powder
1/2 teaspoon baking soda
1/2 teaspoon salt
1/2 teaspoon ground cinnamon
2 egg whites
1/3 cup corn syrup
1 teaspoon vanilla extract
1/3 cup raisins

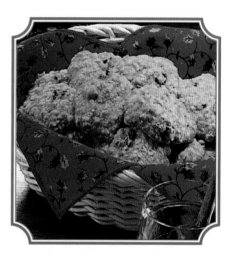

In a medium bowl, combine the first 10 ingredients; mix well. Stir in raisins (dough will be stiff). Drop by tablespoonfuls onto baking sheets coated with nonstick cooking spray. Bake at 375° for 8-10 minutes or until lightly browned. **Yield:** 2-1/2 dozen.

Exchanges: 1-1/2 Starch

Nutritional Information

Serving Size: 2 cookies
Calories: 110
Sodium: 103 mg
Cholesterol: 0 mg

Carbohydrate: 25 gm
Protein: 2 gm
Fat: trace
Fiber: 1 gm

Apple Nut Bars

Karen Nelson, Sullivan, Wisconsin

For big apple taste packed into a yummy bar, try these. The best part is you don't have to peel the apples...that's a real time-saver.

2 egg whites
2/3 cup sugar
1/2 teaspoon vanilla extract
1/2 cup all-purpose flour
1 teaspoon baking powder
2 cups chopped unpeeled tart apples
1/4 cup chopped pecans

In a bowl, whisk egg whites, sugar and vanilla for about 1-1/2 minutes. Add flour and baking powder; whisk for 1 minute. Fold in the apples and pecans. Pour into an 8-in. square baking pan coated with nonstick cooking spray. Bake at 350° for 25-30 minutes or until the bars test done. Cool. **Yield:** 1 dozen.

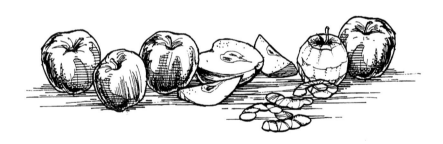

Exchanges: 1 Starch

Nutritional Information

Serving Size: 1 bar
Calories: 92
Sodium: 29 mg
Cholesterol: 0 mg

Carbohydrate: 19 gm
Protein: 1 gm
Fat: 2 gm
Fiber: 1 gm

Cherry-Peach Dumplings

Patricia Frerk, Syracuse, New York

This fruity finale can be made on the stovetop or in an electric skillet right at the dinner table. There's no more convenient way to enjoy a delicious dessert.

1 can (20 ounces) reduced-sugar
   cherry pie filling
1/2 cup water
2 tablespoons lemon juice
1/2 teaspoon ground cinnamon
1/4 teaspoon ground cloves
1 can (15-1/4 ounces) unsweetened
   peach slices *or* halves, drained
1 egg
Skim milk
1-1/2 cups reduced-fat biscuit/
   baking mix
Additional cinnamon, optional
8 tablespoons nonfat whipped
   topping

In a 10-in. skillet, combine the first five ingredients. Add peaches; bring to a boil. Place egg in a 1-cup measuring cup; add enough milk to measure 2/3 cup. Place biscuit mix in a bowl; stir in milk mixture with a fork just until moistened. Drop by eight spoonfuls over top of boiling fruit. Simmer, uncovered, for 10 minutes; cover and simmer 10 minutes longer or until dumplings test done. Sprinkle with cinnamon if desired. Serve warm with whipped topping. **Yield:** 8 servings.

Exchanges: 1-1/2 Fruit, 1 Starch

Nutritional Information

Serving Size: 1/8 recipe
Calories: 188
Sodium: 288 mg
Cholesterol: 27 mg

Carbohydrate: 38 gm
Protein: 4 gm
Fat: 3 gm
Fiber: 1 gm

Soft Gingersnaps

Shonna Lee Leonard, Lower Sackville, Nova Scotia

These soft, cake-like spice cookies are delightfully old-fashioned, which makes it hard to believe they're low in fat.

1-1/2 cups all-purpose flour
1/2 cup whole wheat flour
2 teaspoons baking soda
1 teaspoon ground cinnamon
1 teaspoon ground cloves
1 teaspoon ground ginger
1/4 teaspoon salt
Egg substitute equivalent to 2 eggs
1/2 cup sugar
1/4 cup packed brown sugar
1/4 cup vegetable oil
1/4 cup molasses

In a mixing bowl, combine the flours, baking soda, cinnamon, cloves, ginger and salt. Combine the egg substitute, sugars, oil and molasses; mix well. Add to dry ingredients; mix well. Drop by teaspoonfuls 2 in. apart onto baking sheets coated with nonstick cooking spray. Bake at 350° for 8-10 minutes or until cookies spring back when lightly touched. Cool on pans for 5 minutes before removing to wire racks to cool completely. **Yield:** 3 dozen.

MOLASSES SECRETS. The robust flavor of dark molasses makes it perfect for a classic recipe like gingersnaps. Before measuring molasses, lightly coat the measuring cup with nonstick cooking spray. That way, the molasses will slide right out.

Exchanges: 1/2 Starch, 1/2 Fat

Nutritional Information

Serving Size: 1 cookie
Calories: 63
Sodium: 94 mg
Cholesterol: trace

Carbohydrate: 11 gm
Protein: 1 gm
Fat: 2 gm
Fiber: trace

Cantaloupe Sherbet

Rolanda Crawford, Abilene, Texas

*I depend on this recipe often in summer. You can find me in
the kitchen early in the day preparing it. Then we
sit outside under the evening Texas sky and enjoy every spoonful!*

1 medium ripe cantaloupe
**1 can (14 ounces) nonfat sweetened
   condensed skim milk**
2 tablespoons honey

Cut cantaloupe in half; discard seeds. Peel and slice cantaloupe; cut into large pieces. Place in a blender container. Add milk and honey; cover and blend until smooth. Pour into a freezer-proof container. Freeze overnight or until firm. **Yield:** 9 servings.

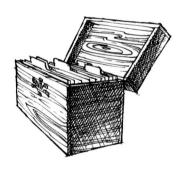

Exchanges: 1 Starch, 1 Fruit

Nutritional Information

Serving Size: 1/2 cup
Calories: 159
Sodium: 58 mg
Cholesterol: 3 mg

Carbohydrate: 36 gm
Protein: 4 gm
Fat: trace
Fiber: trace

Chocolate Mousse with Strawberries

Kim Marie Van Rheenen, Mendota, Illinois

*Everyone in our family savors this simple tempting dessert.
Our young son, who is diabetic, loves this mousse as
"frosting" over angel food cake, too.*

**1 package (1.4 ounces) instant
sugar-free chocolate fudge
pudding mix
1 cup cold skim milk
1-3/4 cups light whipped topping
Whole fresh strawberries**

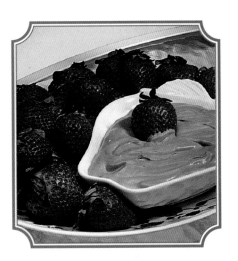

In a mixing bowl, beat pudding and milk
until blended, about 2 minutes. Fold in
whipped topping. Serve with strawberries
for dipping. **Yield:** 2-1/2 cups.

Exchanges: 1 Fruit

Nutritional Information

Serving Size: 2 tablespoons dip
  plus 4-5 large strawberries
Calories: 57
Sodium: 67 mg
Cholesterol: trace

Carbohydrate: 11 gm
Protein: 1 gm
Fat: 1 gm
Fiber: 3 gm

Banana Graham Dessert

Kathy Baker, Hamilton, Georgia

This creamy dessert is reminiscent of the old-fashioned banana pudding Grandma used to serve. It's a nice dish to make in advance.

1 package (1.5 ounces) instant sugar-free vanilla pudding mix
2-3/4 cups cold skim milk
1 cup (8 ounces) nonfat sour cream
12 reduced-fat graham crackers
2 large firm bananas, sliced

In a mixing bowl, beat pudding mix and milk on low speed for 2 minutes. Fold in sour cream. Let stand for 5 minutes. In a 3-qt. bowl, layer a third of the graham crackers, bananas and pudding mixture. Repeat layers twice. Refrigerate. **Yield:** 9 servings.

BANANA BASICS. Bananas are one fruit that continues to ripen after being picked. Green bananas are unripe and need to ripen a few days before using. Ripe bananas should have a nice yellow color with green tips and just a few brown spots.

Exchanges: 1/2 Starch, 1/2 Skim Milk, 1/2 Fruit

Nutritional Information

Serving Size: 1/2 cup
Calories: 139
Sodium: 295 mg
Cholesterol: 4 mg

Carbohydrate: 27 gm
Protein: 6 gm
Fat: 1 gm
Fiber: 1 gm

Sherbet Cake Roll

Karen Edland, McHenry, North Dakota

(ALSO PICTURED ON FRONT COVER)

This light and easy cake roll can be prepared year-round, but it's especially nice in the heat of summer. I like to have this dessert in the freezer ready to serve to unexpected company.

1 package (14-1/2 ounces) one-step angel food cake mix
1/2 gallon sherbet of your choice

Coat two 15-in. x 10-in. x 1-in. baking pans with nonstick cooking spray; line pans with waxed paper and spray the paper. Prepare cake mix according to package directions; spread batter into prepared pans. Bake at 375° for 18-22 minutes or until the cake springs back when lightly touched. Cool in pans for 10 minutes. Turn each cake onto a linen towel dusted with confectioners' sugar. Remove waxed paper; trim off dry edges. Roll up each cake in the towel, starting with a narrow end. Cool on a wire rack. When cooled, unroll cakes; spread each with 4 cups sherbet. Roll up carefully; place seam side down on aluminum foil.

Wrap securely; freeze until firm, about 6 hours. Remove from the freezer 15 minutes before serving. Cut into 1-in. slices. **Yield:** 20 servings.

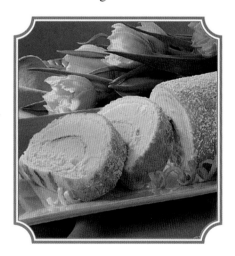

Exchanges: 2 Starch, 1/2 Fat

Nutritional Information

Serving Size: 1 slice
Calories: 186
Sodium: 187 mg
Cholesterol: 5 mg

Carbohydrate: 42 gm
Protein: 3 gm
Fat: 2 gm
Fiber: trace

Old-Fashioned Rice Pudding

Sandra Melnychenko, Grandview, Manitoba

This comforting dessert is a wonderful way to end any meal. As a girl, I always waited eagerly for Mom to serve up the first heavenly bite.

4-1/2 cups skim milk
1/2 cup uncooked long grain rice
1/3 cup sugar
1/2 cup raisins
  1 teaspoon vanilla extract
Ground cinnamon, optional

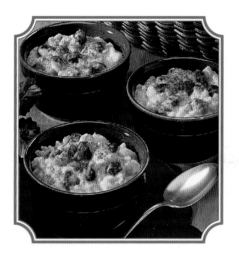

In a saucepan, combine milk, rice and sugar; bring to a boil over medium heat, stirring constantly. Pour into a 1-1/2-qt. baking dish coated with nonstick cooking spray. Cover and bake at 325° for 45 minutes, stirring every 15 minutes. Add raisins and vanilla; cover and bake for 15 minutes. Sprinkle with cinnamon if desired. Serve warm or chilled. Store in the refrigerator. **Yield:** about 6 servings.

Exchanges: 1 Starch, 1 Skim Milk, 1/2 Fruit

Nutritional Information

Serving Size: 1/6 recipe
Calories: 205
Sodium: 102 mg
Cholesterol: 4 mg

Carbohydrate: 43 gm
Protein: 8 gm
Fat: trace
Fiber: 1 gm

Raspberry Angel Food Cake

Christine Wallat, Greenfield, Wisconsin

Fresh sweet raspberries add a special touch to ordinary angel food cake. Each delicious slice is so colorful and attractive.

10 egg whites
1-1/4 teaspoons cream of tartar
1 teaspoon vanilla extract
1/2 teaspoon almond extract
1/2 cup sugar
1 cup cake flour
2 cups fresh raspberries

In a mixing bowl, beat egg whites until frothy; beat in cream of tartar until soft peaks form. Add the extracts. Gradually beat in sugar until stiff, scraping bowl occasionally. Sift flour over beaten whites; sprinkle with berries. Gently fold flour and raspberries into batter until well mixed. Pour into an ungreased 10-in. tube pan. Bake at 325° for 40-45 minutes or until lightly browned and entire top appears dry. Immediately invert cake pan; cool completely, about 1 hour. **Yield:** 16 servings.

BUYING RASPBERRIES. Look for brightly colored, plump raspberries that have a fresh scent. Avoid soft, shriveled or moldy berries. A half-pint yields about 1 cup.

Exchanges: 1/2 Starch, 1/2 Fruit

Nutritional Information

Serving Size: 1 slice
Calories: 75
Sodium: 35 mg
Cholesterol: 0 mg

Carbohydrate: 15 gm
Protein: 3 gm
Fat: trace
Fiber: 1 gm

Crustless Pumpkin Pie

Thelia Busse, Cresco, Pennsylvania

Here's a treat that makes a festive meal complete.

**1 can (15 ounces) solid-pack
  pumpkin
1 can (12 ounces) evaporated skim
  milk
Egg substitute equivalent to 2 eggs
  2 egg whites
Sugar substitute equivalent to 3/4
  cup sugar***
  **1 teaspoon ground cinnamon
  1/4 teaspoon ground allspice
  1/4 teaspoon ground ginger
  1/8 teaspoon salt
  1/2 cup reduced-fat graham cracker
    crumbs
  8 tablespoons light whipped topping
Additional cinnamon, optional**

In a mixing bowl, combine the pumpkin, milk, egg substitute, egg whites and sugar substitute; beat until smooth. Add the spices and salt; beat until well mixed. Stir in graham cracker crumbs. Pour into a 9-in. pie plate coated with nonstick cooking spray. Bake at 325° for 50-55 minutes or until a knife inserted near the center comes out clean. Cool. Garnish with a dollop of whipped topping and sprinkling of cinnamon if desired. Store in the refrigerator. **Yield:** 8 servings. ***Editor's Note:** Sweet 'N' Low or Sweet One are recommended for baking.

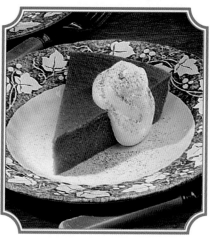

Exchanges: 1 Starch, 1/2 Skim Milk

Nutritional Information

Serving Size: 1 slice
Calories: 109
Sodium: 299 mg
Cholesterol: 2 mg

Carbohydrate: 21 gm
Protein: 5 gm
Fat: 2 gm
Fiber: 2 gm

Almond Spice Cookies

Crystal Landolt, Calgary, Alberta

When my family has the taste for something sweet, this is the recipe I usually reach for. Everyone unanimously declares them delicious!

1/2 cup margarine, softened
3/4 cup sugar
Egg substitute equivalent to 1 egg
1/2 teaspoon almond extract
1-1/4 cups all-purpose flour
1/4 teaspoon *each* ground
    cinnamon, nutmeg and cloves
1/4 teaspoon baking powder
Pinch salt
1/2 cup chopped almonds

In a mixing bowl, cream margarine and sugar; add egg substitute and extract. Combine dry ingredients; add to the creamed mixture. Stir in almonds. Drop by rounded teaspoonfuls onto baking sheets coated with nonstick cooking spray. Bake at 350° for 9-11 minutes or until edges are golden brown. Remove to wire racks to cool. **Yield:** 5 dozen.

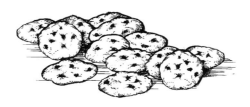

Exchanges: 1 Fat, 1/2 Starch

Nutritional Information

Serving Size: 2 cookies
Calories: 78
Sodium: 35 mg
Cholesterol: trace

Carbohydrate: 9 gm
Protein: 1 gm
Fat: 4 gm
Fiber: trace

Sugar-Free Pineapple Pie

Ethel Lou Haley, Mayfield, Kentucky

Graham cracker crumbs, pudding mix and crushed pineapple gives this tasty pie just the right amount of sweetness. It's easy to double the recipe for a crowd.

**1 cup graham cracker crumbs
(about 16 squares)
1/4 cup margarine, melted
1 package (1 ounce) instant
sugar-free vanilla pudding mix
1 cup (8 ounces) nonfat sour cream
1 can (20 ounces) unsweetened
crushed pineapple, drained
Sugar substitute equivalent to 2
teaspoons sugar**

Combine crumbs and margarine; press into the bottom and up the sides of a 9-in. pie plate. Bake at 350° for 8-10 minutes; cool. In a bowl, combine pudding mix and sour cream; mix well. Stir in pineapple and sugar substitute. Spread into crust. Refrigerate at least 3 hours. **Yield:** 8 servings.

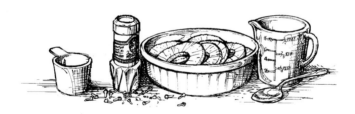

Exchanges: 1-1/2 Fat, 1 Starch, 1/2 Fruit

Nutritional Information

Serving Size: 1 slice
Calories: 178
Sodium: 318 mg
Cholesterol: 3 mg

Carbohydrate: 26 gm
Protein: 3 gm
Fat: 7 gm
Fiber: 1 gm

Sugarless Heart Cookies

Becky Jones, Akron, Ohio

Here's a wonderful treat, even for those not watching sugar intake. It's fun to try new tastes by changing the flavor of the gelatin.

3/4 cup margarine, softened
1 package (.3 ounce) sugar-free mixed fruit gelatin
Egg substitute equivalent to 1 egg
1 teaspoon vanilla extract
1-3/4 cups all-purpose flour
1/2 teaspoon baking powder

In a mixing bowl, cream margarine and gelatin. Beat in egg substitute and vanilla. Add flour and baking powder; mix well. Refrigerate for 1 hour. Roll out on a lightly floured board to 1/4-in. thickness. Cut with a 1-1/4-in. cookie cutter. Place on ungreased baking sheets. Bake at 400° for 6-7 minutes or until bottoms are lightly browned and cookies are set. Cool on wire racks. **Yield:** 6 dozen.

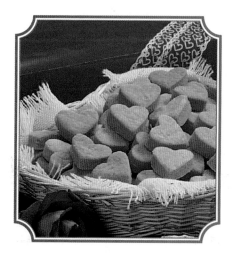

Exchanges: 1/2 Starch, 1/2 Fat

Nutritional Information

Serving Size: 2 cookies
Calories: 55
Sodium: 48 mg
Cholesterol: trace

Carbohydrate: 5 gm
Protein: 1 gm
Fat: 3 gm
Fiber: trace

Diabetic Orange Cookies

Ginette Martino, Deltona, Florida

These good-for-you cookies have a wonderful citrus flavor and just the right amount of natural sweetness. You'll find they appeal to all palates.

1-1/2 cups all-purpose flour
1 teaspoon baking powder
Sugar substitute equivalent to 3/4 cup sugar*
2 teaspoons grated orange peel
1/4 teaspoon salt
1/8 teaspoon ground nutmeg
1/2 cup margarine spread (70% vegetable oil)
1/3 cup chopped raisins
Egg substitute equivalent to 1 egg
2 tablespoons orange juice

In a medium bowl, combine the first six ingredients; mix well. Cut in margarine until mixture resembles coarse crumbs. Stir in raisins. Add egg substitute and orange juice; mix well. Drop by teaspoonfuls onto baking sheets coated with nonstick cooking spray. Flatten with a fork dipped in flour. Bake at 375° for 13-15 minutes. **Yield:** 30 cookies. ***Editor's Note:** Sweet 'N' Low or Sweet One are recommended for baking.

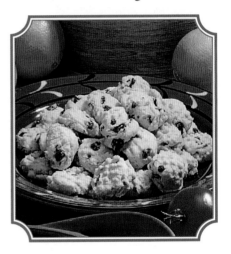

Exchanges: 1 Starch, 1/2 Fat
Nutritional Information

Serving Size: 2 cookies
Calories: 112
Sodium: 122 mg
Cholesterol: trace

Carbohydrate: 15 gm
Protein: 2 gm
Fat: 6 gm
Fiber: 1 gm

Strawberry Dessert

Marcille Meyer, Battle Creek, Nebraska

This recipe yields a large volume, so it's great to take to a potluck or family gathering. The cool, creamy pudding pairs well with the angel food cake and strawberries.

1 loaf (10-1/2 ounces) angel food cake, cubed
1 package (1 ounce) instant sugar-free vanilla pudding mix
1 cup cold skim milk
2 cups fat-free sugar-free vanilla ice cream, softened
1 package (.3 ounce) sugar-free strawberry gelatin
1 cup boiling water
1 cup cold water
1 package (20 ounces) frozen unsweetened strawberries, partially thawed and sliced

Place cake cubes in an ungreased 13-in. x 9-in. x 2-in. baking dish. In a mixing bowl, beat pudding mix and milk on low for 1-1/2 minutes. Add ice cream; beat on low for 1 minute. Pour over cake; chill. Dissolve gelatin in boiling water. Add cold water and strawberries; mix until partially set. Spoon over pudding layer. Cover and refrigerate overnight. **Yield:** 24 servings.

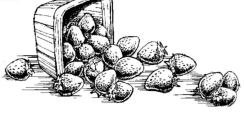

Exchanges: 1 Starch

Nutritional Information

Serving Size: 1/24 recipe
Calories: 61
Sodium: 129 mg
Cholesterol: trace

Carbohydrate: 14 gm
Protein: 2 gm
Fat: trace
Fiber: 1 gm

Pecan Cookies

Bonnie Jolly, Bailey, Colorado

*Around our house, we especially enjoy these
slightly sweet nutty cookies for a midday snack
But my family also likes them for a nice breakfast treat.*

1-1/2 cups whole wheat flour
1/2 cup all-purpose flour
1 teaspoon baking powder
2 tablespoons quick-cooking oats
1/2 cup margarine
3/4 cup finely chopped pecans
1/2 cup packed brown sugar
1/4 to 1/2 cup skim milk

In a large bowl, combine flours and baking powder; stir in oats. Cut margarine into pieces; cut into flour mixture until well mixed. Add pecans and brown sugar; mix well. Stir in enough milk with a fork to form a stiff paste. Turn onto a floured surface; knead lightly until smooth. Roll out on a floured surface to 1/4- to 1/8-in. thickness. Cut with a 1-1/2-in. round cookie cutter. Place on baking sheets coated with nonstick cooking spray. Bake at 375° for 10 minutes or until lightly browned. Cool on wire racks. **Yield:** about 7-1/2 dozen.

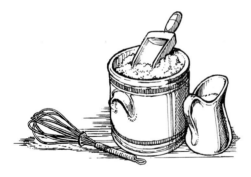

Exchanges: 1/2 Starch, 1/2 Fat
Nutritional Information

Serving Size: 2 cookies
Calories: 59
Sodium: 27 mg
Cholesterol: trace

Carbohydrate: 7 gm
Protein: 1 gm
Fat: 3 gm
Fiber: 1 gm

Condiments

You and your family will relish the
added flavor these sauces, salsas, dressings
and toppings give your favorite foods.

Strawberry Salsa

Jean Giroux, Belchertown, Massachusetts

This deliciously different salsa is versatile, fresh-tasting and colorful. People are surprised to see a salsa made with strawberries, but it's excellent over grilled chicken and pork

1 pint fresh strawberries, diced
4 plum tomatoes, seeded and
  diced
1 small red onion, diced
1 to 2 medium jalapeno
  peppers, minced*
Juice of 1 lime
  2 garlic cloves, minced
  1 tablespoon olive *or*
  vegetable oil

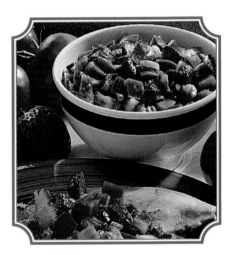

In a bowl, combine strawberries, tomatoes, onion and peppers. Stir in lime juice, garlic and oil. Cover and refrigerate for 2 hours. Serve with cooked poultry or pork or as a dip for tortilla chips. **Yield:** 4 cups. ***Editor's Note:** When cutting or seeding hot peppers, use rubber or plastic gloves. Avoid touching your face.

Exchanges: 1/2 Fruit
Nutritional Information

Serving Size: 1/2 cup
Calories: 38
Sodium: 4 mg
Cholesterol: 0 mg

Carbohydrate: 5 gm
Protein: 1 gm
Fat: 2 gm
Fiber: 1 gm

Low-Fat Gravy

Mary Fry, Cedar Rapids, Iowa

With this special sauce, folks on restricted diets don't have to pass on the gravy. Instead, they can say, "Please pass the gravy!" Now you can smother slices of turkey without guilt.

1/2 cup finely chopped onion
1/2 cup finely chopped fresh
  mushrooms
2 tablespoons chopped fresh
  parsley
2 cups reduced-sodium beef *or*
  chicken broth, *divided*
2 tablespoons cornstarch
Pinch pepper

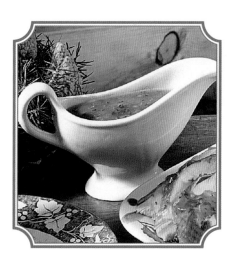

In a saucepan, saute onion, mushrooms and parsley in 1/4 cup broth until vegetables are tender. Combine cornstarch, pepper and 1/2 cup of broth; stir until smooth. Add to pan with the remaining broth. Bring to a boil, stirring occasionally; boil for 2 minutes. **Yield:** 2 cups.

SERVING SUGGESTION. Serve this succulent gravy over slices of Garlic Rosemary Turkey (recipe on page 165).

Exchanges: Free food

Nutritional Information

Serving Size: 1/4 cup
Calories: 23
Sodium: 28 mg
Cholesterol: 1 mg

Carbohydrate: 4 gm
Protein: 1 gm
Fat: trace
Fiber: trace

Rhubarb Relish

Helen Brooks, Lacombe, Alberta

I remember eating this tangy relish at my grandmother's over 50 years ago. My mother made it for years and now my daughters make it. It complements any meat.

12 cups finely chopped fresh *or* frozen rhubarb
1 large onion, chopped
3/4 cup cider vinegar
1/4 teaspoon salt
1 teaspoon ground cloves
1 teaspoon ground cinnamon
1/2 teaspoon ground allspice
1/4 teaspoon paprika
Sugar substitute equivalent to 1 cup sugar

In a large saucepan, combine the first eight ingredients. Bring to a boil. Reduce heat and simmer for about 2 hours or until mixture thickens, stirring occasionally. Stir in sugar substitute. Pour into jars. Refrigerate or freeze in covered containers. **Yield:** 4 pints.

RELISH RHUBARB YEAR-ROUND. To enjoy the taste of rhubarb out of season, cut rhubarb into 1-inch chunks and freeze in heavy-duty plastic bags for up to 9 months.

Exchanges: Free Food

Nutritional Information

Serving Size: 1/4 cup
Calories: 13
Sodium: 2 mg
Cholesterol: 0 mg

Carbohydrate: 3 gm
Protein: trace
Fat: 0 gm
Fiber: 1 gm

Cranberry Pear Chutney

Carol Bricker, Tempe, Arizona

My husband is a diabetic who likes to round out a meal with this lovely sauce. The fruity ingredients in this sugar-free treat give it a natural sweetness.

2 cups fresh *or* frozen cranberries
3/4 cup frozen unsweetened
   apple juice concentrate, thawed
1 pear, peeled and cubed
1/2 cup raisins

In a saucepan, bring cranberries and concentrate to a boil. Cook and stir for 5 minutes. Add pear and raisins; cook and stir until berries pop and pear is tender, about 5-7 minutes. Pour into a serving bowl; refrigerate overnight. **Yield:** 2 cups.

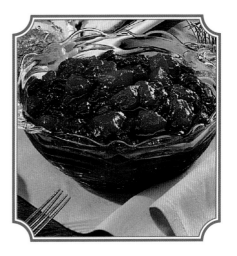

Exchanges: 1 Fruit

Nutritional Information

Serving Size: 1/4 cup
Calories: 58
Sodium: 4 mg
Cholesterol: 0 mg

Carbohydrate: 15 gm
Protein: trace
Fat: trace
Fiber: 2 gm

Cardamom Yogurt Sauce

Geraldine Grisdale, Mt. Pleasant, Michigan

*With a creamy texture and hint of spice, this
delicious sauce really complements a variety of fruit.*

1 egg
1/4 cup orange juice
1 tablespoon honey
1 teaspoon ground
  cardamom
1 carton (8 ounces) plain nonfat
  yogurt

In a small saucepan, combine egg, orange juice, honey and cardamom. Cook over medium heat, stirring constantly, until mixture reaches 160° and thickens, about 5 minutes. Cook and stir 2 minutes longer. Cool for 20 minutes; fold in yogurt. Cover and refrigerate for at least 1 hour. Serve over oranges, bananas and apples or fruit of your choice. **Yield:** 1-1/4 cups.

MOUTH-WATERING CARDAMOM. Cardamom has a cool, peppery taste that complements many foods, especially sweets. Since a little cardamom goes a long way in recipes, buy in smaller quantities so it doesn't have to be stored for a long time.

Exchanges: 1/2 Skim Milk

Nutritional Information

Serving Size: 1/4 cup
Calories: 59
Sodium: 47 mg
Cholesterol: 43 mg

Carbohydrate: 8 gm
Protein: 4 gm
Fat: 1 gm
Fiber: trace

Zesty Salsa

Sharon Lucas, Raymore, Missouri

*The addition of olives makes this salsa a little different from
other varieties. You can seed the jalapeno peppers if you like.
But if your family likes salsa with some "heat", leave them in.*

8 medium tomatoes, chopped
3/4 cup sliced green onions
1/3 cup finely chopped fresh
   cilantro *or* parsley
1/3 cup chopped onion
2 small jalapeno peppers, finely
   chopped* (seeded if desired)
1 can (2-1/4 ounces) sliced ripe
   olives, drained
3-1/2 teaspoons fresh lime juice
1 tablespoon cider vinegar

1 tablespoon vegetable oil
1 to 2 teaspoons chili powder
1 to 2 teaspoons ground cumin
1 teaspoon garlic powder
1 teaspoon dried oregano
1/4 teaspoon salt

Combine all ingredients in a large bowl.
Cover and refrigerate overnight. **Yield:** 12
servings. ***Editor's Note:** When cutting or
seeding hot peppers, use rubber or plastic
gloves. Avoid touching your face.

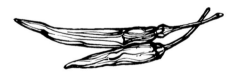

Exchanges: 1 Vegetable, 1/2 Fat

Nutritional Information

Serving Size: 1/12 recipe
Calories: 41
Sodium: 105 mg
Cholesterol: 0 mg

Carbohydrate: 6 gm
Protein: 1 gm
Fat: 2 gm
Fiber: 1 gm

Italian Salad Dressing

George Greenauer, Spencerport, New York

*As a diabetic who likes salads, I was tired of
plain vinegar and oil topping the greens.
So I came up with this tongue-tingling dressing!*

1/4 cup vegetable oil
1/4 cup cider *or* red wine vinegar
1 garlic clove, minced
1 teaspoon finely chopped
onion
1/2 teaspoon ground mustard
1/2 teaspoon celery seed
1/2 teaspoon paprika
1/4 teaspoon Italian seasoning
Sugar substitute equivalent to 2
to 4 teaspoons sugar

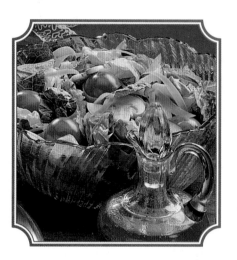

Combine all ingredients in a jar with a
tight-fitting lid; shake well. Refrigerate
overnight. **Yield:** 2/3 cup.

Exchanges: 2 Fat

Nutritional Information

Serving Size: 2 tablespoons
Calories: 82
Sodium: trace
Cholesterol: 0 mg

Carbohydrate: 1 gm
Protein: trace
Fat: 9 gm
Fiber: trace

Apricot-Nut Spread

Ruth Stenson, Santa Ana, California

This nice and tart spread can add extra-special flavor to homemade muffins and biscuits, especially when the baked goodies are fresh from the oven.

1 package (6 ounces) dried apricots
1/2 cup water
1 package (8 ounces) light cream cheese, cubed and softened
1/4 cup chopped walnuts

Soak apricots in water overnight. Drain, reserving 2 tablespoons liquid. Place apricots and reserved liquid in a blender or food processor. Cover and process for about 10 seconds. Add cream cheese; process just until blended. Add walnuts and blend until mixed. Store in the refrigerator. **Yield:** 2 cups.

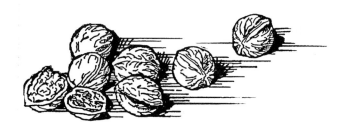

Exchanges: 1/2 Fruit, 1/2 Fat

Nutritional Information

Serving Size: 2 tablespoons
Calories: 70
Sodium: 53 mg
Cholesterol: 5 mg

Carbohydrate: 10 gm
Protein: 2 gm
Fat: 2 gm
Fiber: 1 gm

Spicy Corn and Black Bean Relish

Gail Segreto, Elizabeth, Colorado

This relish can be served as a salad or as a garnish for a Southwestern meal—it's especially good with chicken.

2-1/2 cups fresh *or* frozen corn, cooked and drained
1 can (15 ounces) black beans, rinsed and drained
3/4 to 1 cup chopped seeded Anaheim chili peppers*
1/8 to 1/4 cup chopped seeded jalapeno peppers*
1/4 cup vinegar
2 tablespoons vegetable oil
1 tablespoon Dijon mustard
1 teaspoon chili powder
1 teaspoon ground cumin
3/4 teaspoon salt-free seasoning blend
1/2 teaspoon pepper

In a large bowl, combine corn, beans and peppers. Combine remaining ingredients in a small bowl; pour over corn mixture and toss to coat. Refrigerate. **Yield:** 8 servings. ***Editor's Note:** When cutting or seeding hot peppers, use rubber or plastic gloves. Avoid touching your face.

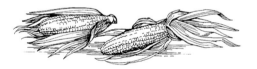

Exchanges: 1 Starch, 1 Fat

Nutritional Information

Serving Size: 1/8 recipe
Calories: 128
Sodium: 295 mg
Cholesterol: 0 mg

Carbohydrate: 19 gm
Protein: 5 gm
Fat: 4 gm
Fiber: 5 gm

Low-Fat Blue Cheese Dressing

Tracey Baysinger, Salem, Missouri

*You'll never miss the fat in this full-flavored dressing!
The recipe comes from a chef at a California resort.*

**1 cup (8 ounces) fat-free
cottage cheese**
**1 cup (8 ounces) plain nonfat
yogurt**
2 tablespoons chopped onion
1 garlic clove, minced
**1 tablespoon crumbled blue
cheese**

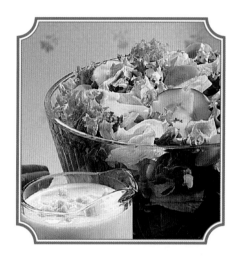

In a blender or food processor, combine cottage cheese, yogurt, onion and garlic; cover and process until smooth. Stir in blue cheese. Store, covered, in the refrigerator. **Yield:** 1-3/4 cups.

Exchanges: Free Food

Nutritional Information

Serving Size: 2 tablespoons
Calories: 23
Sodium: 80 mg
Cholesterol: 1 mg

Carbohydrate: 2 gm
Protein: 3 gm
Fat: trace
Fiber: trace

Stewed Rhubarb

Caroline Simpson, Fredericton, New Brunswick

*This is my husband's favorite way to enjoy rhubarb.
He has it for breakfast over cereal or for dessert,
either plain or over fat-free sugar-free ice cream.*

**5 to 6 cups chopped fresh *or* frozen
   rhubarb
1 cup water
1/2 teaspoon ground cinnamon
Sugar substitute equivalent to 3/4 cup**

In a saucepan, bring rhubarb and water
to a full rolling boil. Add cinnamon; return to a boil. Reduce heat and simmer
10 minutes or until sauce reaches desired
consistency. Stir in sugar substitute. Cool.
Yield: 5 cups.

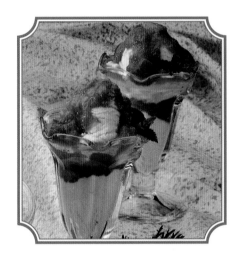

Exchanges: Free Food

Nutritional Information

Serving Size: 1/2 cup

Calories: 13

Sodium: 2 mg

Cholesterol: 0 mg

Carbohydrate: 3 gm

Protein: 1 gm

Fat: trace

Fiber: 1 gm

Tomato-Garlic Dressing

Diane Hyatt, Renton, Washington

I've served this salad dressing many times when having company over for dinner and everyone just loves it. The recipe has been in my files for so long, I forgot where it originally came from.

2 cups fat-free mayonnaise
1 teaspoon lemon juice
1 teaspoon garlic powder
2 medium tomatoes, cubed

Combine all ingredients in a food processor or blender. Cover and process until smooth. Refrigerate. **Yield:** about 3 cups.

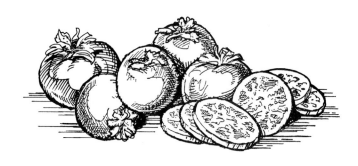

Exchanges: Free Food

Nutritional Information

Serving Size: 2 tablespoons
Calories: 16
Sodium: 141 mg
Cholesterol: 0 mg

Carbohydrate: 3 gm
Protein: trace
Fat: trace
Fiber: trace

Cranberry Salsa

Arline Roggenbuck, Shawano, Wisconsin

Wisconsin grows an abundance of cranberries and celebrates the harvest with many cranberry festivals. This unique salsa is easy, different and good! Try it with pork or turkey.

2 cups fresh *or* frozen cranberries
2 cups water
Sugar substitute equivalent to 1/2 cup sugar
1/4 cup minced fresh cilantro *or* parsley
2 to 4 tablespoons chopped jalapeno peppers*
1/4 cup finely chopped onion
2 tablespoons grated orange peel
1/2 teaspoon salt-free seasoning blend
1/4 teaspoon pepper

In a saucepan, bring cranberries and water to a boil; boil for 2 minutes. Drain. Stir in sugar substitute until dissolved. Add cilantro, peppers, onion, orange peel, seasoning blend and pepper. Mix well. Cool and refrigerate. **Yield:** 2 cups. ***Editor's Note:** When cutting or seeding hot peppers, use rubber or plastic gloves. Avoid touching your face.

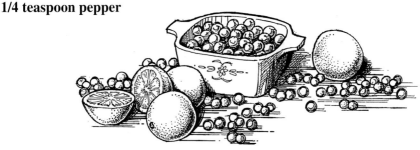

Exchanges: Free Food
Nutritional Information

Serving Size: 1/4 cup
Calories: 18
Sodium: 2 mg
Cholesterol: 0 mg

Carbohydrate: 4 gm
Protein: trace
Fat: trace
Fiber: 1 gm

Fresh Peach Sauce

Dottye Wolf, Rolla, Missouri

*I like to make my breakfast table as pretty as possible.
This peach sauce adds a warm golden color to the table and
terrific flavor to pancakes, waffles and French toast.*

1/2 cup water
2 teaspoons cornstarch
Dash ground nutmeg
1 cup sliced peeled fresh peaches
Sugar substitute equivalent to 3
tablespoons sugar
1/8 to 1/4 teaspoon almond extract

In a saucepan, bring the water, cornstarch and nutmeg to a boil; boil for 1 minute. Add peaches. Bring to a boil; boil 1-2 minutes longer. Remove from the heat; stir in sugar substitute and extract. **Yield:** 1 cup.

PEELING A PEACH. To easily remove the skin from a peach, try this: Dip a peach into boiling water for 20 to 30 seconds; remove with a slotted spoon and immediately plunge into a bowl of ice water. Remove the skin with a paring knife.

Exchanges: 1/2 Fruit

Nutritional Information

Serving Size: 1/4 cup
Calories: 23
Sodium: trace
Cholesterol: 0 mg

Carbohydrate: 6 gm
Protein: trace
Fat: trace
Fiber: 1 gm